THE NEW LIFE LIBRARY

HOMEOPATHY

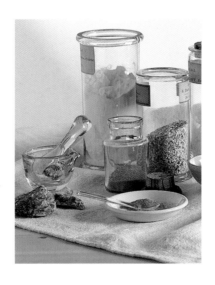

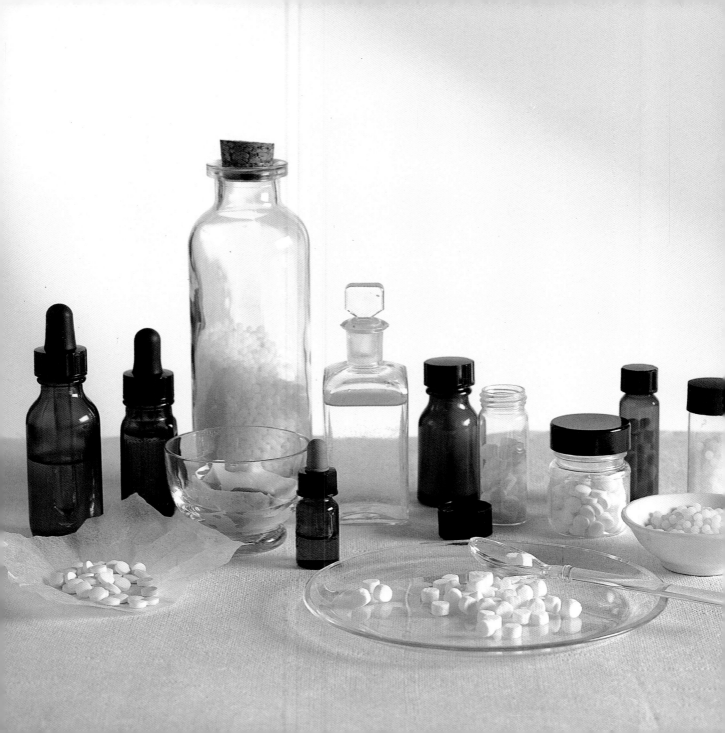

THE NEW LIFE LIBRARY

HOMEOPATHY

SIMPLE REMEDIES FOR NATURAL HEALTH

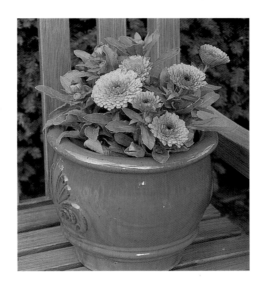

ROBIN HAYFIELD

LORENZ BOOKS

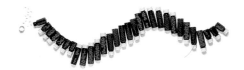

First published by Lorenz Books

Lorenz Books is an imprint of
Anness Publishing Limited
Hermes House
88-89 Blackfriars Road
London SE1 8HA

This edition published in the USA by Lorenz Books, Anness Publishing Inc.,
27 West 20th Street, New York, NY 10011; (800) 354-9657

ISBN 1 85967 626 X

A CIP catalogue record for this book is available from the British Library

Publisher: Joanna Lorenz
Editorial Manager: Helen Sudell
Designer: Bobbie Colgate Stone
Photographer: John Freeman
Stylist: Fanny Ward
Models: Andrea Newland, Stephen Sillett,
Mary Scott, Dominic Scott, Stephen Bartholomew

Publisher's Note:
The reader should not regard the recommendations, ideas and techniques expressed and described in this book as substitutes for the advice of a qualified medical practitioner or other qualified professional. Any use to which the recommendations, ideas and techniques are put is at the reader's sole discretion and risk.

3 5 7 9 10 8 6 4 2

Printed and bound in China

CONTENTS

INTRODUCTION

THE NAME "HOMEOPATHY" was coined by Samuel Hahnemann from two Greek words meaning "similar suffering", or "like cures like". This is a natural principle that has been known for thousands of years, but it was not until the end of the 18th century that Hahnemann (1755-1843), a brilliant German doctor and chemist, started on the course of study and experimentation that led to the development of modern homeopathy. Appalled by the savage medical practices of the day, he formulated a system of healing that was not only extremely safe, but scientifically based. His philosophy of disease and its cure through natural processes has changed very little from that day to this.

The principle of like curing like, or "the law of similars", as it is sometimes called, decrees that if a substance can cause harm to a healthy person in large doses, it also has the potential to cure the same problem in tiny doses by stimulating the body's own natural energy, enabling it to heal itself.

The law is best illustrated by example. In the 19th century it was a custom among German women to take the herb Valerian regularly as a stimulant. The practice was much abused and caused overtaxing of the nervous system. Yet, given in minute doses, Valerian relaxes the nervous system, and calming the mind is one of homeopathy's main remedies for insomnia.

The doses used in homeopathy are so small that they cannot be acting directly on the physical body. Hahnemann considered that they acted dynamically: that the energy of the remedy stimulated the natural healing energy of the body, if it was in a state of disharmony, in order to return to its former healthy state.

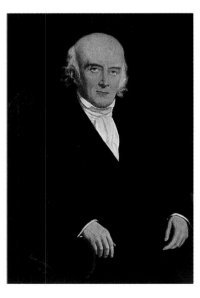

Above: Samuel Hahnemann (1755-1843), the first homeopath.

Right: There are many chemical compounds that are used for homeopathic remedies.

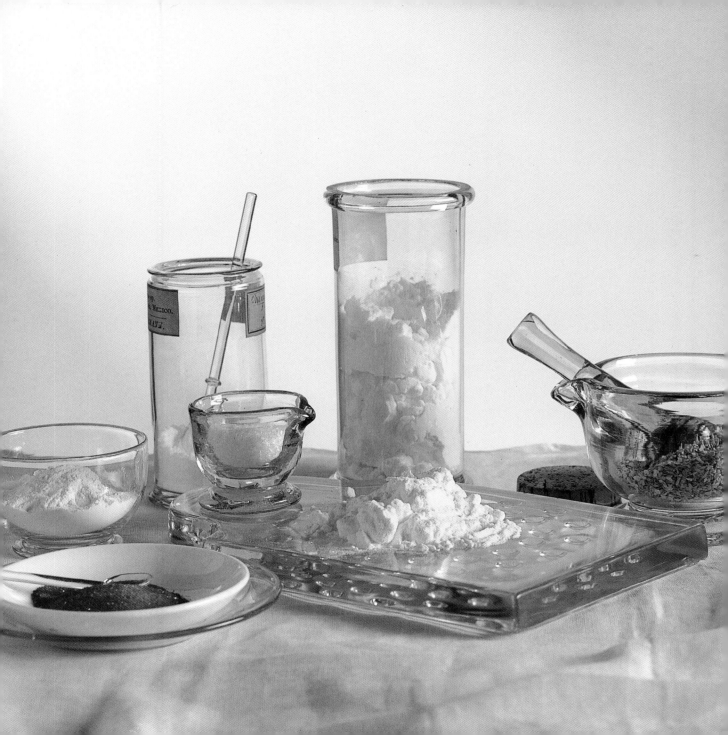

HOW HOMEOPATHY WORKS

Homeopathy is not only an energy medicine but is also holistic. Homeopaths believe that the body is much more than the sum of its various parts and that the whole person should be treated. The mind, the emotions and all the various organs are interconnected. It would be unwise to treat one part without considering the whole person.

ENERGY WITHIN

The mechanics of this interconnection are extremely complex and almost impossible to understand in any detail. Luckily, in homeopathy we don't have to. We trust the process. Underlying the intricate physical and mental systems of the body is a refined and subtle system of energy, which is self-regulating and works efficiently almost all the time. We see it in action when we become ill. We feel unwell, have unpleasant symptoms, then we usually get better whether we take medicines or not. The body does its own healing, although it may sometimes need support when its own natural sources of healing energy are depleted or unbalanced.

THE HEALING PROCESS

The healing process can be compared to running a car. Modern cars are so efficient that, provided you maintain them properly, give them the right fuel and drive them sensibly, problems seldom arise. Then one night, you forget to turn the lights off and the next morning the battery is flat and the car incapacitated. The only way to get the car moving again – the only cure – is to get a transfer of energy, in the form of a jump start from the battery of another car. Then all will be well. Homeopathy is a bit like getting a jump start! The energy sources are the remedies, used in accordance with the law of similars so that the body can run on all cylinders again.

Above: Sometimes our bodies get stuck in disease, and we need a boost from a homeopathic remedy to get things moving again.

A SAFE THERAPY

Many people turn to homeopathy because of their concerns about orthodox medicine, which is now very drug-orientated. Many drugs are very toxic and the side-effects in susceptible people can be very distressing. Even if the side-effects are not observable, the long-term problems associated with excessive use of drugs are little understood. Modern medicine seldom cures and it does not pretend to. It alleviates and palliates symptoms, and "manages" the illness, but since it addresses only the symptoms and seldom the disease itself, the results are often unsatisfactory. It is not holistic – consultants tend to be specialists in small parts of the system, ignoring the other parts.

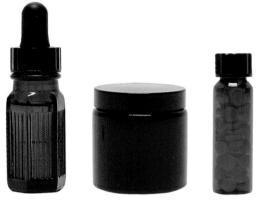

Above: Remedies usually come in tablet form. But they can also be made up into creams and tinctures.

THE HOLISTIC PRINCIPLE

Homeopathy is safe to use and does not treat the removal of symptoms as an end in itself. Symptoms are considered as signs of distress or adjustment. The correct remedy removes the cause of the problem; the distressing symptoms will then fade away.

Homeopathy takes into account the nature of the person. It individualizes and recognizes that even if two people are diagnosed as having the same illness, they become ill in different ways and will need different remedies to effect a proper cure.

USING HOMEOPATHY

For chronic, or long-term, illnesses, you should consult a professional homeopath who will have had many years of training and subsequent experience. But for acute, non-serious ailments there is much good work that you can do yourself, with a small number of remedies and a book like this.

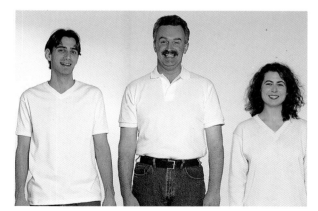

Above: Homeopathy individualizes. Different people are treated with different remedies for the same ailment.

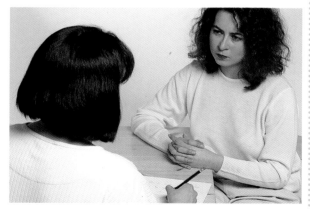

Above: You cannot treat chronic problems yourself. For these go and consult a qualified homeopath.

THE NATURE OF DISEASE: WHY WE GET ILL

We become ill when our energy is depleted or when we are out of harmony. The word "disease" should perhaps more accurately be written "dis-ease", indicating that we are not at ease. For a disease to be cured it is not necessary to give it a name. To cure homeopathically depends on an analysis of the symptoms. There is usually no need for a diagnosis, for it is said that there are no diseases, only "dis-eased" people.

SYMPTOMS

Except in life-threatening situations, symptoms – painful or distressing though they may be – are not the primary problem. They reflect a picture of how the system is making adjustments to heal itself.

For example, diarrhoea or vomiting is a necessary procedure for the body to rid itself of something it does not want in the quickest most effective way. Pain can be a warning that rest and stillness are immediately required, and it may also be a cry for help.

The intolerable itching of eczema does not specifically mean that you have a skin disease. Rather it means that there is imbalance in your whole system, and your body is pushing the problem to the safest possible place, as far away from the essential organs as possible. The skin is in fact an organ of elimination, and the suppressive use of steroids is not really helpful from a homeopathic point of view.

TREATING THE WHOLE PERSON

To cure well, it is necessary to see the whole picture and understand the person thoroughly. We are all individuals and have different weaknesses and susceptibilities. Some people are very robust and seldom become ill, apart from the odd cold. Others are over-sensitive and become run-down and sick after catching a slight chill or after some emotional upset. For some, their chest is their greatest weakness: every winter cold seems to turn to bronchitis. For others, it

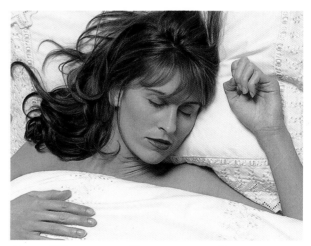

Above: When we get ill, ease turns to dis-ease. Adjustments are needed to restore health.

is their digestion: the slightest unusual change in their diet causes an immediate upset.

Homeopathy acknowledges these differences and adjusts the treatment accordingly. The professional homeopath will prescribe "constitutionally" to try to strengthen the weak areas as well as the whole system.

CAUSES OF ILLNESS

There are many causes of disease. Some are obvious, such as the bruising or shock that follow an accident. A run-down and overworked constitution will probably not escape a winter flu epidemic.

Poor nutrition is another underlying cause. In the

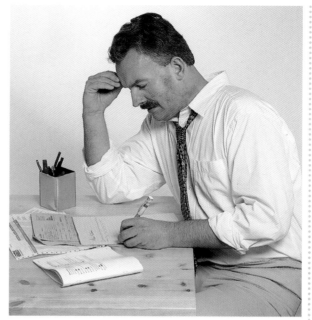

Above: Mental and emotional stress can cause physical problems in the long run.

developed world, most people have enough to eat, but in these days of factory farming and junk food, the quality may not be good. Essential minerals and vitamins are often lacking.

Finally, illness may have an emotional cause. Stress is a major contributor to inner disharmony, which then manifests itself in physical ailments. Grief, fear, worry, depression and loneliness are not compatible with good health.

Homeopathy takes all these factors into account and, if possible, tries to mitigate them and strengthen the sufferer to be able to cope better with them.

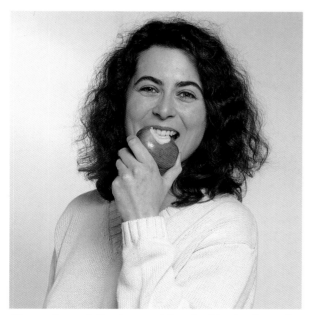

Above: A good diet is essential to health. Apples and other fruit are especially good for you.

THE VITAL FORCE AND THE IMMUNE SYSTEM

With so much battering from within and without, it may seem a wonder that we are not all permanently ill. Of course, many people are. Although many of the acute infectious diseases of the past have ceased to be a serious problem, their places have been taken by today's chronic diseases. Never has there been so much cancer and heart disease, eczema and asthma, or digestive problems such as irritable bowel disease. Our immune systems are overstretched in combating these problems.

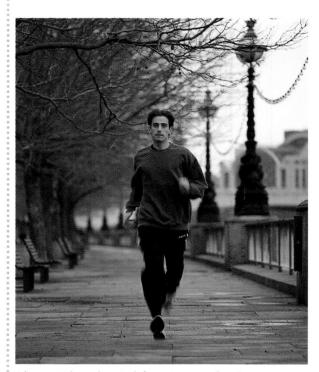

Above: When the vital force is in perfect harmony, you will feel you can do anything!

THE IMMUNE SYSTEM

It is all too easy to ignore the incredible adaptability and intelligence of the immune system, which appears to make heroic efforts to keep us up and running despite considerable adversity. Hahnemann named this intelligence the "vital force". He described it as "the spirit-like force which rules in supreme sovereignty". It has also been described as "the invisible driver", overseeing the checks and balances of the immune system which operate to keep us in the best possible health.

THE VITAL FORCE AT WORK

Most of the time we are not aware of this balancing process – it is quite automatic and pre-programmed through our genetic inheritance. We can observe it in action when we contract an acute illness (one that arises suddenly) such as a fever or a cough. What we may not always realize is that the fever is necessary to burn up infection, and that the cough is there to prevent accumulation of mucus in the lungs. If the vital force cannot aid the curative process with acute diseases, it is forced to deal with

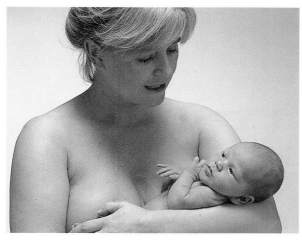

Above: We are all born with a vital force that oversees our health.

the problem through chronic disease (ones that are not self-limiting but are persistent and of long duration). Then it may need outside help.

THE SYMPTOM PICTURE

In its attempt to cure a disease, the vital force causes the body to produce symptoms. Homeopaths call this the symptom picture. These symptoms not only reflect what is going on inside but can also indicate what outside help or extra energy is required.

While it is true to say that in homeopathy we do not treat symptoms but the person who has them, we are nevertheless extremely interested in the symptoms. For it is through careful observation of the complete symptom picture that we will discover which remedy is required. In acute ailments, which are the subject of this book, the vital force will eventually cure, given

time. But by giving it a helping hand through noting what it needs via the symptoms and then giving the body an "energy fix" with the indicated remedy, the process can be speeded up considerably.

For example, suppose there is a flu epidemic and two children in a family catch it. The first child catches it very suddenly, literally overnight, and he develops a very high fever, with a red face and a dry burning heat all over his body. The second child's symptoms come on very slowly over several days. This child's fever is much lower, but she is shaky and shivery and her muscles ache all over. It's the same flu for both children, but the vital force has produced completely different symptoms. Each child therefore needs to be responded to in a different way. The homeopath will understand this and give the first child the remedy Belladonna and the second child Gelsemium.

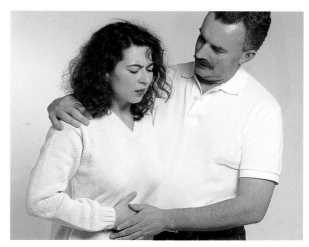

Above: All symptoms have meaning. Pain is a warning that there is disorder in the system.

REMEDIES AND THEIR SOURCES

The remedies used in homeopathy are derived from many sources. The majority are prepared from plants, but many minerals are also used and a few remedies are prepared from insect and snake poisons and other toxic substances. There is no need to be alarmed about their poisonous origins, for homeopathic remedies have been so diluted that no possible danger remains.

MAKING REMEDIES

The law of similars shows that the most powerful poisons can be turned into equally powerful remedies. Hahnemann discovered and used about a hundred remedies. About two thousand have now been described, but most professional homeopaths use only a fraction of that number.

To turn a substance into a remedy, so that the energy is tamed and harnessed, is an involved process usually carried out by a homeopathic pharmacy. The process itself is called potentization, and consists of two main procedures in alternation: dilution and succussion (or vigorous shaking).

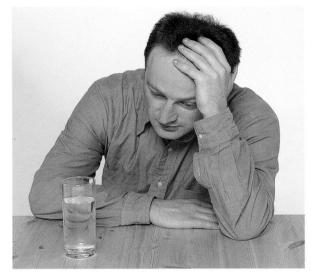

Above: In homeopathy, all symptoms are taken into account in finding the correct remedy.

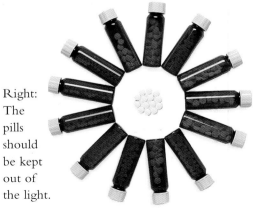

Right: The pills should be kept out of the light.

When you buy a remedy you will notice a number after its name, commonly 6, but also other numbers rising in a scale: 30, 200, 1M (1,000). Sometimes a "c", standing for centesimal (one hundredth) is written after the number. The number represents the potency, or the number of times the remedy has been diluted and succussed.

PREPARING HOMEOPATHIC REMEDIES

A remedy is prepared by dissolving a tincture of the original material – usually in alcohol. On the centesimal scale, the 6th potency means that the original substance has been diluted six times, each time using a dilution of one part in a hundred. This results in a remedy that contains only one part in a million million of the source material. Barely any molecules of the original substance will be present at this dilution, and if the potency is increased to 12c, there will be none left at all. Yet the greater the potency (or number of dilutions), the greater the power of the remedy seems to be. It may seem puzzling that homeopathy can possibly work at such a dilution, but you need to remember that it is an energy medicine and not primarily a physical one.

Between each dilution, the remedy is succussed. The phial (vial) in which it is being prepared is shaken

TISSUE SALTS

The 19th-century German doctor, Wilhelm Schussler, identified 12 vital minerals, or "tissue salts", essential to health. According to his theory, many diseases are associated with a deficiency of one or more of these substances, but can be cured by taking the tissue salts in minute doses, singly or in various combinations.

vigorously or banged a number of times. This is very important and ensures the release and transfer of energy from the original substance to the remedy. When the potentization is complete the remedy is preserved in alcohol, and a few drops can be added to a bottle of milk-sugar pills or a cream. This is called medicating the remedy, which is now ready to use.

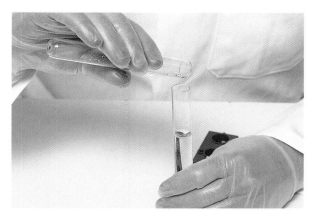

Above: The potentization of a remedy is carried out through a process of dilution and succussion (vigorous shaking and banging).

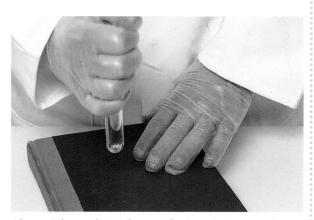

Above: The traditional way of succussing a remedy was to use an old leather-bound bible on which to bang the test tube.

PROVINGS AND SYMPTOMS

Almost all homeopathic remedies have been "proved", or tested, although practitioners gain additional knowledge of them from clinical experience. In a proving, a remedy is tested on a group of healthy people over a period of time, until they develop symptoms. Neither the supervisor nor the group should know what remedy they are proving. This is a true double blind test, conducted on scientific principles. The symptoms that the provers develop are tabulated and collated until a complete symptom picture is obtained. Now we know what the remedy can cure.

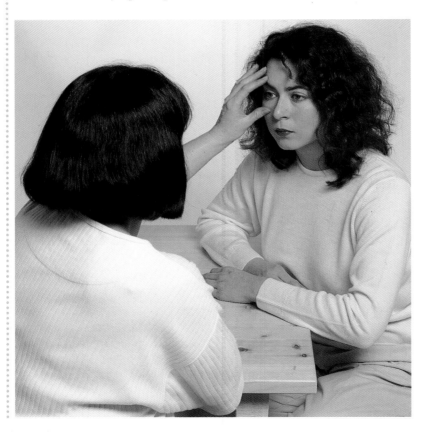

MATERIA MEDICA

Once proved, remedies can be used for all time. They do not go in and out of fashion. Almost all of Hahnemann's original hundred remedies are constantly in use today. Remedy pictures are detailed in large volumes called Materia Medica. Because so many symptoms for so many remedies have been proved over the last two hundred years, no homeopath could possibly remember them all. They are listed in another detailed book called The Homeopathic Repertory, which in effect is an index to the Materia Medica. These two books between them should cover almost all symptoms.

Left: In homeopathy, physical examinations are seldom necessary, but bright, sparkling eyes are a sign of good health.

CHOOSING THE CORRECT REMEDY

With a knowledge of Materia Medica, the homeopath is equipped to match the symptoms of the person with the symptom picture of the remedy. This is called finding the similimum (or similar).

PUTTING TOGETHER THE SYMPTOM PICTURE

Finding the correct remedy is like trying to arrange a perfect marriage. If the two partners are compatible, success is almost certain. If the remedy is a good match to the symptoms, the patient is going to feel a good deal better, the natural way. The words "I feel better in myself" are like music to the ears of the prescribing homeopath, because it means that the natural healing processes have been stimulated successfully, even if some of the physical symptoms remain. It should be only a short time before they too disappear.

The prescriber is like a detective looking for clues. Apart from the obvious general symptoms, such as fever, headache or a cough, you should note what are called the "modalities" – that is, what aggravates or alleviates the symptoms, or makes the person feel generally better or worse. They could include the need for warmth, or cool air, sitting up or lying down. Notice whether the person is thirsty or sweaty; whether the tongue is coated and the state of the breath. What kind of pain is it: throbbing, stitching or sudden stabs of intense agony?

Do the symptoms have an obvious cause? Did they arise after an emotional shock, or after catching a chill in a cold wind? Did they arise dramatically and suddenly in the middle of the night, or have they developed in rather a nondescript way over a number of days?

It is also very important to note the person's state of mind. For example, irritable people who just want to be left alone may need quite different remedies from those who want to be comforted and are easily consoled.

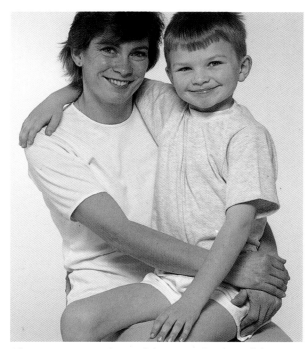

Above: Even members of the same family will have different susceptibilities to illness and react differently.

When and How to Use Remedies

Many minor and self-limiting acute problems can be treated safely at home with a basic first-aid kit. However, for more serious long-term ailments, or if you feel out of your depth and really worried — especially if young children or old people are ill — seek help from your own homeopath or your doctor.

PROFESSIONAL HOMEOPATHS

Access to professional homeopaths is much easier nowadays and they can often do wonderful things for persistent and chronic disease. Qualified practitioners will have completed three or four years' training.

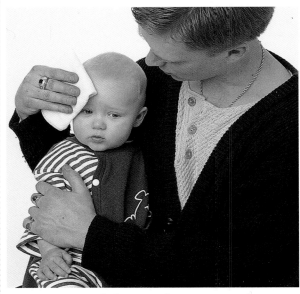

Above: You may feel unsure about treating very young children, but homeopathy usually works brilliantly on them, and can be safely used from birth.

HOMEOPATHIC FIRST-AID

What you are trying to do is help the body help itself. Sometimes there may not be a great deal you can do — a well-established cold is going to mean several days of suffering whether you intervene or not. In other cases, the sooner you act, the better: for instance, if you give Arnica (either in pill form, or rubbed-in cream if appropriate) immediately after a bad fall for the bruising and shock, the results will be very impressive.

You can often limit the duration or intensity of suffering, such as in fever, sepsis (pus-forming bacteria), pain, indigestion and many other conditions. Moreover, there will be many satisfying times when the problem is aborted or cured altogether.

Once you see an improvement, the vital force needs no further help and you can stop the remedy. You will do no harm if you don't, but there is no point in giving more energy than needed. In homeopathy "less is more".

GIVING THE REMEDY

The 6th and 30th potencies are most useful for home use. As a rough rule of thumb, use a 6c three or four times a day, or a 30c once or twice daily until symptoms improve. One pill at a time is all that is necessary and there is no need to reduce the dosage for children.

Sometimes the symptoms may change after giving a remedy, so that a new picture emerges. You then need to find a new remedy to fit the new picture. If the situation improves, or the picture is unclear, watch and wait. Only intervene if you feel you need to.

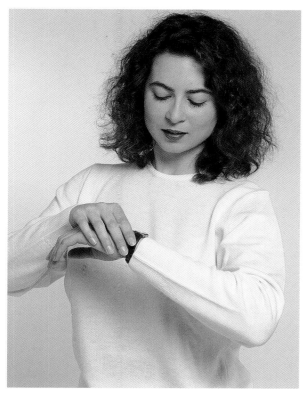

Above: After placing a remedy on your tongue, suck it for about 30 seconds before crunching.

In serious situations such as a high fever or after an accident, you can give a remedy every half-hour if necessary. You can't overdose in acute situations and if you don't get a good reaction within a day or overnight, you may want to consider a second remedy. Never worry about giving the wrong remedy: it will either work or it won't. If it doesn't, you will have done no harm.

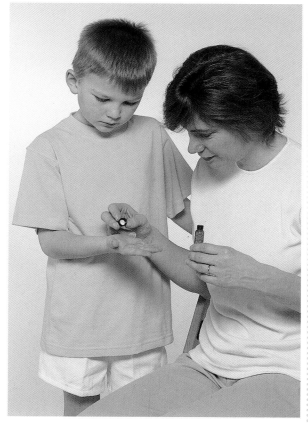

Above: The simplest way to give a child a remedy is to pour one tablet from the cap into the patient's hand and then place it directly into the mouth.

THE HOMEOPATHIC FIRST-AID KIT

It's a good idea to keep a basic first-aid kit in the house so that you are prepared for all emergencies. Many remedies are available from health food shops or some chemists. But there may not be a source near you and it is amazing how many homeopathic situations arise outside shop-opening hours.

OBTAINING REMEDY KITS

You can obtain a remedy kit from a good homeopathic pharmacy. All pharmacies will supply their own kits, or make one up to your own specifications. This can be as big or small as you like.

This book describes 42 remedies. Many of these you may never need, so it would be wise to begin with about half that number: these will cover most common situations. You can then add more remedies as you become more confident and experienced.

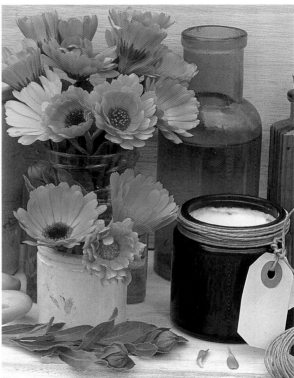

Above: Calendula cream is the best remedy to use on open cuts and sores.

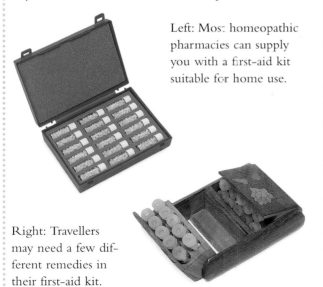

Left: Most homeopathic pharmacies can supply you with a first-aid kit suitable for home use.

Right: Travellers may need a few different remedies in their first-aid kit.

YOUR FIRST-AID KIT SHOULD INCLUDE:

ARNICA CREAM – for bruises

CALENDULA CREAM – for cuts and sores

RESCUE REMEDY TINCTURE – for major emergencies

ECHINACEA TINCTURE – for the immune system

PLUS THESE BOTTLES OF PILLS:

ACONITE – for fevers, coughs and colds

APIS – for bites and stings

ARNICA – for bruising or shock following accidents

ARSENICUM – for digestive upsets, food poisoning

BELLADONNA – for high fever, headache

BRYONIA – for dry coughs and fevers

CHAMOMILLA – for teething, colic

FERRUM PHOS – for colds and flu, anaemia

GELSEMIUM – for flu and anxiety

HEPAR SULPH – for sore throats, infected wounds

HYPERICUM – for injuries

IGNATIA – for grief and emotional upsets

LEDUM – for puncture wounds, bites and stings

LYCOPODIUM – for anxiety, digestive problems

MERCURIUS – for sepsis

NUX VOMICA – for hangovers, nausea, indigestion

PHOSPHORUS – for digestive problems, nosebleeds

PULSATILLA – for ear infections, fevers, eye problems

RHUS TOX – for sprains and strains, rashes

RUTA – for injuries to tendons and bones

RESCUE REMEDY

Although not strictly a homeopathic treatment, Rescue Remedy is one of Dr Edward Bach's Flower Remedies. These flower essences are a series of gentle plant remedies which are intended to treat various emotional states, regardless of the physical disorder. For practical purposes, the Rescue Remedy is the finest treatment available for alleviating symptoms of shock. It is a compound of five of Dr Bach's original remedies, namely Impatiens, Star of Bethlehem (*Ornithogatum umbellatum*), Rock rose (*Cistus*), Cherry plum (*Prunus cerasifera*) and *Clematis vitalba*.

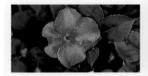

Impatiens.

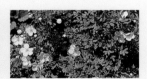

Cherry plum.

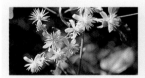

Clematis.

Rock rose.

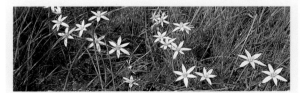

Star of Bethlehem.

REMEDIES FOR COMMON AILMENTS

MANY STRAIGHTFORWARD problems can be treated at home using homeopathy. For each one, a number of remedies are listed on the following pages that are likely to be most helpful. Read the remedy picture carefully and choose the one that seems to make the best "fit" with the symptoms you have observed. When you have selected your remedy, double-check it with the more detailed description in the Materia Medica section towards the end of the book.

HOW TO TAKE THE REMEDY
Once you have chosen the remedy, empty one pill into the cap of the bottle. If more than one lands in the cap, tip the others back into the bottle without touching them.

Drop the pill on to a clean tongue – that is, you should take the remedy at least 10 minutes before or after eating, drinking or cleaning your teeth. The pill should be sucked for about 30 seconds before being crunched and swallowed. Remedies for babies can be crushed to a powder in an envelope and given on a teaspoon.

ECHINACEA
Echinacea angustifolia, or the purple cornflower, is a native American herb. It is a general tonic for the immune system, and is particularly useful to take if you have been feeling run down for a while.

Above: Sympathy and a hug is sometimes the best medicine.

Right: Homeopathy is an exacting science.

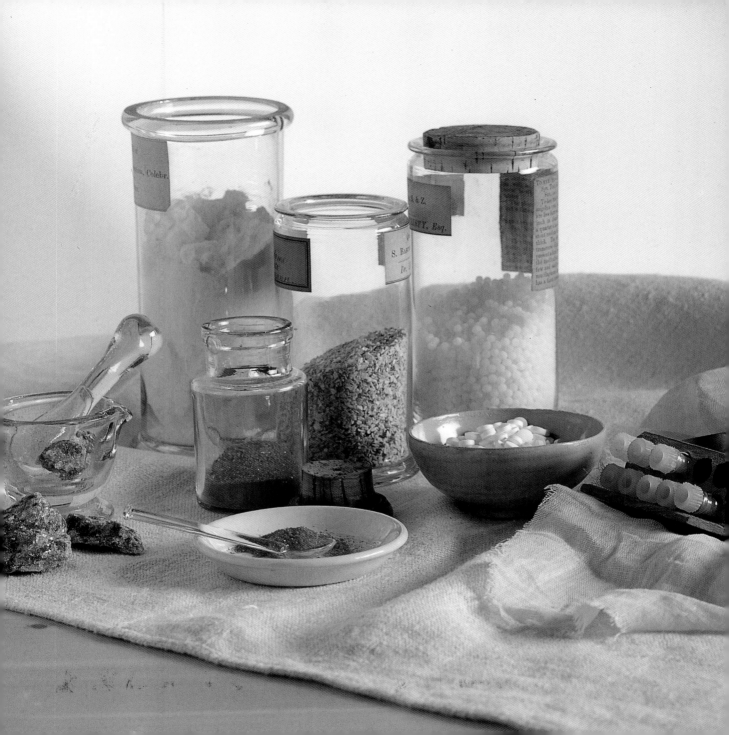

FIRST-AID TREATMENTS

Homeopathic remedies can be used as first-aid treatment in many situations, but serious injuries should always receive expert medical attention. If you are worried, call for help first, then give the appropriate remedy while you wait for help to arrive.

BRUISES

The very first remedy to think of after any injury or accident is *ARNICA*. For local bruising, where the skin is unbroken, apply Arnica cream, and whether you use the cream or not you can give an Arnica pill as often as you think necessary, until the bruising starts to go down. Arnica is also

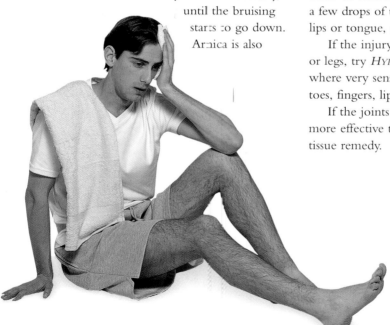

wonderful in cases of shock. If the person is dozy (woozy) or unconscious, crush the remedy first and place the powder directly on the lips.

Where there is serious shock, or in any real emergency, use *RESCUE REMEDY*. This can be used either alone or with Arnica in cases of physical trauma. Place a few drops of the Rescue Remedy straight on to the lips or tongue, every few minutes if necessary.

If the injury results in pains shooting up the arms or legs, try *HYPERICUM*. This remedy is very useful where very sensitive areas have been hurt, such as the toes, fingers, lips and ears.

If the joints or bones have been hurt, *RUTA* may be more effective than Arnica, which is more of a soft tissue remedy.

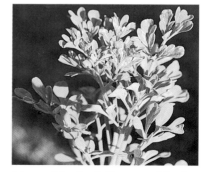

Above: The herb Rue, used in the remedy Ruta.

Above: After any injury or shock, the first remedy to think of is Arnica.

24

CUTS, SORES AND OPEN WOUNDS

The first priority is to clean the area gently but thoroughly to remove any dirt. If the wound is very deep, it may need stitches and you should seek medical help. Once the wound is clean, gently apply some *CALENDULA* cream. *HYPERCAL* cream, which is a mixture of Calendula and *HYPERICUM*, will do equally well. If necessary, add a dressing to keep the wound clean.

PUNCTURE WOUNDS

Such injuries can arise from animal or insect bites, pins, needles and nails, or from standing on a sharp instrument such as a garden fork (rake).

If the wound becomes puffy and purple and feels cold, yet the pain is eased by cold compresses, *LEDUM* is the best remedy. If there are shooting pains, which travel up the limbs along the tracks of the nerves, then *HYPERICUM* should be used.

SPRAINS AND STRAINS

For general muscle strains, resulting from lifting heavy weights or excessive physical exercise such as aerobics or long hikes over hilly countryside, *ARNICA* will almost always be extremely effective. For deeper injuries where the joints are affected, as a result of a heavy fall or a strong football tackle, use *RUTA*.

For even more severe sprains, especially to the ankles or wrists, where the pain is agony on first moving the joint but eases with gentle limbering up, *RHUS TOX* should be very helpful.

For injuries where the slightest movement is extremely painful and hard pressure eases the pain, use *BRYONIA*.

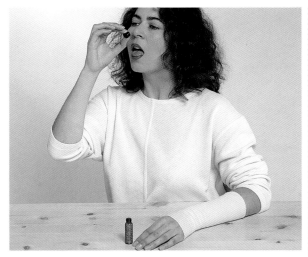

Above: Rhus tox can be a very good remedy for sprains, especially to the ankles or wrists.

FRACTURES

Once a broken bone has been set, use *SYMPHYTUM* daily, night and morning, for at least three weeks. This will not only ease the pain but also speed up the knitting of the bones.

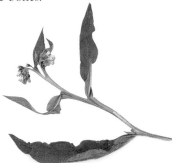

Above: Comfrey, used in the remedy Symphytum.

BURNS

Severe burns need urgent medical assistance: do not delay, especially in the case of children and babies.

For minor burns and scalds, *CALENDULA* or *HYPERCAL* cream is very soothing, especially if applied straight away. If the pain remains, or the burn is more severe, take one pill of the remedy *CANTHARIS* every few hours until the pain eases. If shock is involved or you have a hysterical child, also use *ARNICA* (in pill form) and/or *RESCUE REMEDY*.

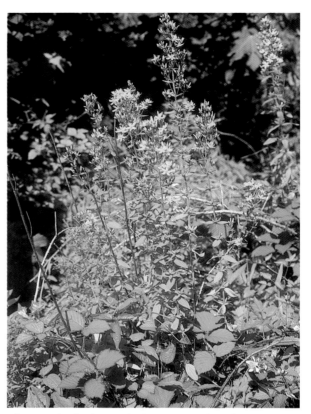

Above: The herb St John's Wort, used in the remedy Hypericum.

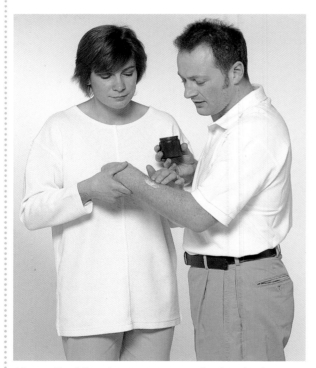

Above: For bites that come up as a bruise, Arnica cream can be very effective.

BITES AND STINGS

For minor injuries, apply *CALENDULA* or *HYPERCAL* cream. If the wound looks bruised, use *ARNICA*, either as a cream or in pill form. If the wound becomes very swollen and looks red and puffy, use *APIS*.

For injuries to sensitive areas, such as fingers, especially if shooting pains can be felt, *HYPERICUM* will be a useful remedy. *LEDUM* would be preferable if the wound is puffy and cold to the touch, yet is helped by cold compresses.

TRAVEL SICKNESS
Many people get seasick in rough weather and some, especially children, are also air-sick or car-sick. The symptoms are usually eased by the remedy *COCCULUS*.

FEAR OF FLYING
For sheer terror, use *ACONITE* and/or *RESCUE REMEDY* before you go to the airport and then as often as you need to during the flight. If you shake with anxiety, try *GELSEMIUM*.

If the problem is more a question of claustrophobia, the fear of being trapped in a narrow space, *ARG NIT* should be very useful.

VISITS TO THE DOCTOR OR DENTIST
For any surgery or dental work where bruising and shock to the system are involved, you cannot go wrong with *ARNICA*. Take one pill just before

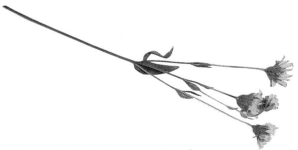

Above: The herb Arnica, used in the remedy of the same name.

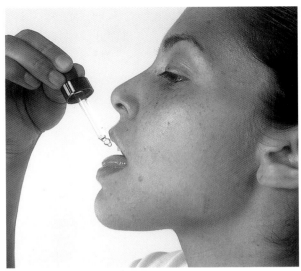

Above: Rescue Remedy can be wonderful in states of extreme anxiety, and in emotional shock.

treatment and one pill three times a day for as long as you need it.

For wounds that are slow to heal, or where there is sepsis, apply *CALENDULA* or *HYPERCAL* cream. If there are injuries to the nerves, the symptoms of which may be shooting pains along the nerve tracks, *HYPERICUM* can be helpful.

Where post-operative bleeding is a problem, such as after a tooth extraction, *PHOSPHORUS* should stop it. Phosphorus is also very useful for that post-anaesthetic "spacey" feeling that won't go away. Sometimes, persistent nausea may remain. *IPECAC* can be wonderful in such circumstances.

For pre-dentist nerves, *ARG NIT* and *GELSEMIUM* are two of the best remedies.

TREATMENTS FOR COLDS AND FLU

Most colds, unless nipped in the bud, take their course and should clear up in a week or so. Flu can be much more debilitating, but a good remedy can often ameliorate the symptoms.

COLDS AND FLU

If flu comes on suddenly, often at night and perhaps after catching a chill, with symptoms of high fever and profuse sweating, ACONITE is a good remedy. If the symptoms are similarly sudden and with a high temperature, but with redness, burning heat and a headache, the remedy is more likely to be BELLADONNA.

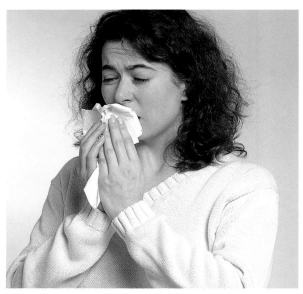

Above: At the first sign of a head cold, try Arsenicum or Allium cepa.

For flu that appears more slowly, accompanied by extreme thirst, irritability and the desire to be left alone, BRYONIA will be very useful.

Probably the most widely used remedy in flu is GELSEMIUM. The most pronounced symptoms are shaking with shivering, aching muscles and general weakness. Where aching bones are prominent, use EUPATORIUM.

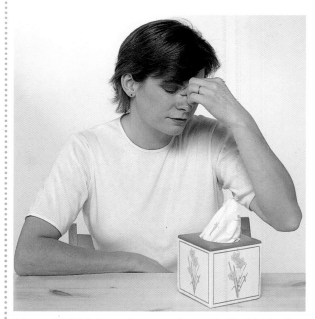

Above: Kali bich can be a good remedy for blocked sinuses where there is pain and a green stringy discharge.

28

For head colds with sneezing and an acrid nasal discharge, *ALLIUM CEPA* or *ARSENICUM* should help. If the sinuses are also affected and there is a lot of yellow-green mucus which appears in globules or looks sticky and stringy, use *KALI BICH*.

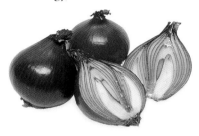

Above: The red onion is used to make the remedy Allium cepa.

For a general tonic, both during and after the flu, when symptoms are not very well defined and there is general malaise, try *FERRUM PHOS*.

COUGHS AND CROUP
For very harsh, dry, violent coughs, which may appear suddenly and may be worse at night, use *ACONITE*. For a hard, dry painful cough, which seems to be helped by holding the chest very tightly and also by long drinks of cold water, use *BRYONIA*.

For deep-seated, dry, spasmodic coughs that may end in retching or even vomiting, use *DROSERA*. Painful, barking coughs, which produce thick yellow-green mucus, may be helped by *HEPAR SULPH*. For coughs that are suffocating and sound like a saw going through wood, try *SPONGIA*. Where there is a lot of mucus seemingly trapped in the chest, try *ANT TART*.

Croup is a horrible sounding dry cough that affects small children. The main remedies are *ACONITE*, *HEPAR SULPH* and *SPONGIA*. Try each in turn, if it is difficult to differentiate between the symptoms.

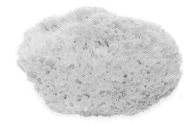

Above: Natural sponge.

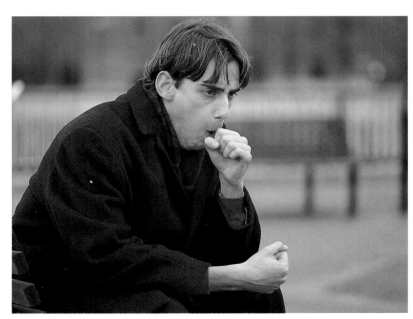

Above: Harsh, dry coughs are often helped by Bryonia.

29

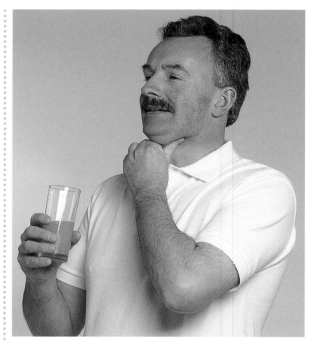

Above: There are many remedies for sore throats. Check the symptoms carefully before deciding.

SORE THROATS

If a sore throat starts suddenly, often during the night, perhaps following a chill and accompanied by a high temperature, try *ACONITE*. If the throat burns and throbs painfully and looks very red, it may be eased by *BELLADONNA*.

For a sore throat that looks very swollen and puffy, with a stinging pain, try *APIS*. *HEPAR SULPH* can be used for an extremely painful throat that feels as if there is a fish bone stuck in it, making it very hard to swallow.

If the sore throat feels worse on the left side and swallowing liquids is particularly painful, use *LACHESIS*. Use *LYCOPODIUM* if the throat is worse on the right side or the pain moves from right to left; warm drinks may be comforting.

For a sore throat accompanied by offensive breath and saliva, plus sweatiness and thirst, try *MERCURIUS*. For throats that look dark and red and feel as if a hot lump has got stuck inside, try *PHYTOLACCA*.

FEVERS

Fevers, particularly in children, whose temperatures may be quite high, may seem alarming, but it should

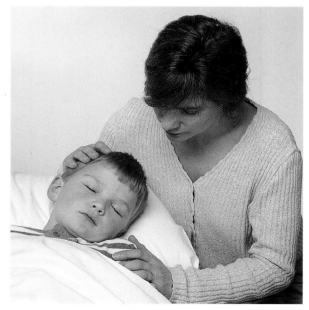

Above: The most useful remedies at the start of a high fever in children are Aconite and Belladonna.

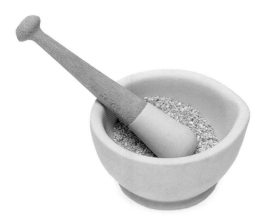

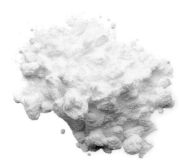

The lime of oyster shells (above) and flowers of sulphur (right) are heated together to make the remedy for Hepar sulph.

be remembered that they are the body's natural response to dealing with and burning up infection.

The two main remedies for high fevers that appear suddenly and often dramatically are *ACONITE* and *BELLADONNA*. There is usually thirst and sweat present in the Aconite picture, while Belladonna cases will be characterized by a dry skin, redness and a throbbing pain in the affected area.

If the fever appears more slowly and the person is irritable, wants to be left alone and is very thirsty for long drinks of cold water, try *BRYONIA*. For flu-like fevers, with shivering, weakness and aching muscles, use *GELSEMIUM*. *FERRUM PHOS* can be used in milder fevers, with no particularly distinctive symptoms.

PULSATILLA is really useful in children's fevers, where the child is very emotional, clingy and weepy and wants to be held and comforted.

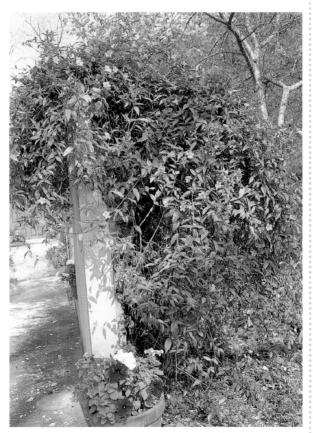

Above: The North American plant, Gelsemium.

EASING EAR INFECTIONS

Acute earaches are most common in young children. They need to be treated quickly, as an infection within the middle ear can be both painful and damaging. Speedy home help can be very useful, but get medical help if the earache worsens or persists.

One of the most soothing remedies is *VERBASCUM* oil. Pour a few drops into a warmed spoon, and insert gently into the child's ear.

For sudden and violent pains, accompanied by fever which usually start at night, use *ACONITE*. Where there is a fever with a sudden and violent appearance and the ear throbs and looks very red, *BELLADONNA* will cure it.

For earaches where there is great pain and the child is exceptionally irritable, use *CHAMOMILLA*. *FERRUM PHOS* is indicated where the pain comes on slowly and there are no other particularly distinguishing symptoms. For very painful and sore earaches with some discharge of yellow-green mucus, when the child is also chilly and irritable, use *HEPAR SULPH*. For pains that extend to the throat and sinuses, accompanied by sweating, thirst and bad breath, use *MERCURIUS*.

PULSATILLA suits children who prefer to be kept cool and seem to feel better when they are held and comforted. The earaches may come and go without particular reason.

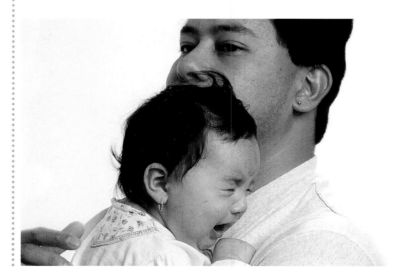

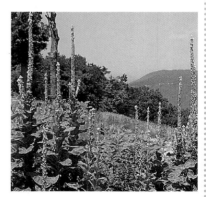

Above: Verbascum.

Left: An effective cure for children's earaches is Verbascum oil.

SOOTHING THE EYES

Overwork, pollutants, viral and bacterial infections can all affect the delicate tissues in and around the eyes. Stress and fatigue tend to aggravate these problems by weakening the immune system's ability to fight off infection.

ACONITE is indicated when the eye feels hot and dry, perhaps after catching a cold in it. It may feel as if a piece of grit is irritating it. *APIS* is a good remedy to use when the eyelids look puffy and swollen and the discomfort is relieved by cold compresses.

For eyes that look red and bloodshot and are over-sensitive to light, *BELLADONNA* is indicated, while *EUPHRASIA* is one of the very best remedies for sore and burning eyes. It can also be used in an eyebath, as it can be obtained in a diluted tincture.

One of the best remedies for styes is *PULSATILLA,* which should be used for eye infections with a sticky yellow discharge.

When treating eye injuries, *SYMPHYTUM* can be used where there has been a direct blow to the eye-ball. For general injuries to the eye, *ARNICA* is often the most helpful remedy to ease the bruising. *LEDUM* will come into its own if, after an injury, the eye is cold and puffy, yet the pain is eased by cold compresses.

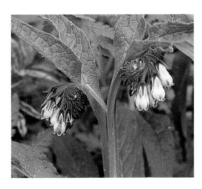

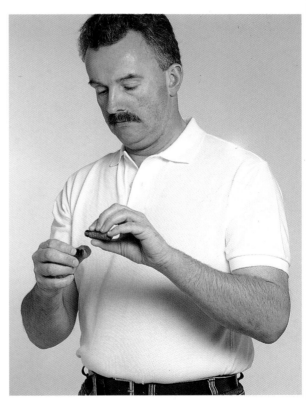

Above: Aconite can be good in some eye infections – but check the symptoms first.

Left: Comfrey, used in the remedy Symphytum.

SETTLING GASTRIC UPSETS

The main symptoms of stomach and intestinal infections are pain, wind (gas), nausea, vomiting or diarrhoea. Bear in mind that vomiting and diarrhoea are natural processes by which the body rids itself quickly of unwanted material, so these symptoms need to be treated only if they are persistent. Such problems can arise at any time and may be due to food poisoning or may just be a reaction to unfamiliar food, perhaps while you are on vacation.

UPSET STOMACH

The great stand-by remedy is *ARSENICUM*. Other symptoms which may accompany diarrhoea or vomiting are excessive weakness, coldness and restlessness. *MAG PHOS* is an excellent remedy for general abdominal cramps which are helped by doubling up and by warmth.

For constant nausea which is unrelieved by vomiting, use *IPECAC*. *NUX VOMICA* is a good remedy for gastric upsets where nothing really seems to happen. Undigested food lies like a dead weight in the stomach – if only it could be vomited, you would feel better.

PHOSPHORUS can be a useful remedy for diarrhoea that runs like a tap, especially if there is a sensation of burning in the stomach. You may crave cold water, but it is vomited up as soon as it has warmed up in the stomach.

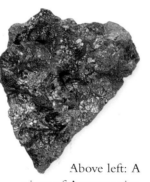

Above left: A piece of Arsenopyrite, containing the metallic mineral arsenic, used in the remedy Arsenicum.

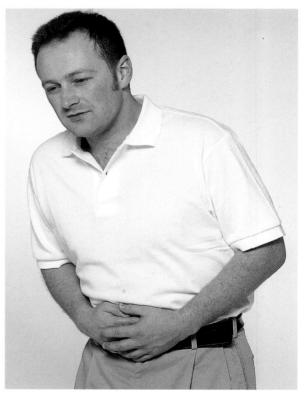

Above: In food poisoning, where there is pain and vomiting or diarrhoea, think of Arsenicum.

INDIGESTION

The symptoms of indigestion are heartburn, wind (gas) and cramping pains. They are usually caused by eating too much or too quickly, especially if you are eating very rich food and drinking alcohol.

The most useful remedy is *NUX VOMICA*. The digestive system seems stuck, heavy and sluggish and the feeling is that you would feel much better if the undigested food would move – up or down or out!

Another remedy that is sometimes helpful is *LYCOPODIUM*. Trapped wind (gas) can cause extreme discomfort. Late afternoon or early evening is often the worst time for this, and the feeling is sometimes accompanied by anxiety. The remedy often works well on people whose gastric system is the weakest part of their constitution.

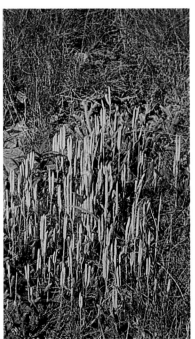

Above: Lycopodium.

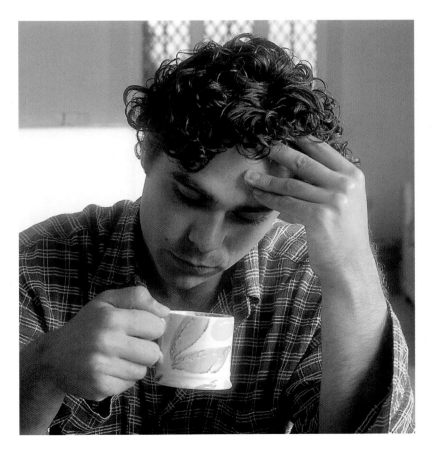

Left: Nux vomica can be a great remedy in indigestion – especially after a good night out!

CALMING BOILS AND ABSCESSES

Sometimes, an area of the skin becomes inflamed and gathers pus. This usually happens around a hair follicle. The build-up of pus can cause acute pain before it comes to a head as a boil or abscess, or until the pus is absorbed by the body.

In the early stages of a boil or abscess, when it looks red and angry and throbs painfully, *BELLADONNA* is often the best remedy. Later when it starts becoming septic (infected) and even more painful as the pus increases, use *HEPAR SULPH.*

If the boil seems very slow in coming to a head, *SILICA* should be used to speed up the process. This remedy is also helpful as a daily tissue salt for unhealthy skin that keeps producing boils. The nails may also be unhealthy, breaking and peeling too easily.

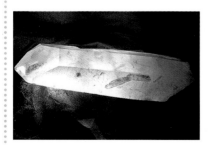

Above: The original proving for Silica was rock crystal.

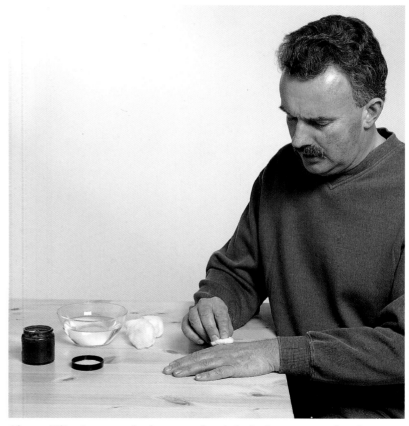

Above: Silica is a remedy that can often help boils come to a head.

RELIEVING TOOTHACHE

There is probably no worse agony than toothache, as the area is so sensitive. In most cases, a visit to the dentist will be essential, but the following remedies may help with the pain in the meantime.

For sudden and violent pains, perhaps precipitated by a cold, *ACONITE* may be helpful. If the area looks very red and throbs violently, *BELLADONNA* should be used. For abscesses, where pus is obviously present and the saliva tastes and smells foul, the best remedy is likely to be *MERCURIUS*. If you are prone to abscesses and your teeth are generally not very strong, *SILICA* should be used to strengthen the system.

For pain that lingers after a visit to the dentist, take *ARNICA* or *HYPERICUM*. If the pain is accompanied by extreme irritability, *CHAMOMILLA* should be used.

HEPAR SULPH is a suitable remedy for extreme septic states (infected areas), where bad temper is a prominent symptom. Another remedy for toothache where there are spasmodic shooting pains is *MAG PHOS*.

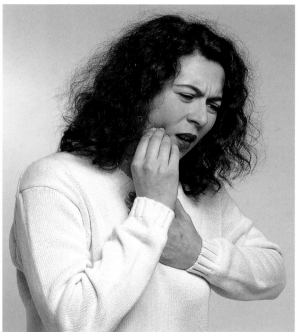

Above: There are several remedies that can help with toothache, but you still need to visit the dentist.

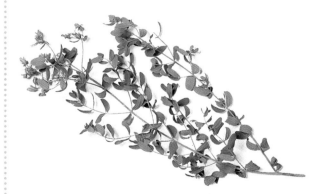

Above: St John's Wort, for the remedy Hypericum.

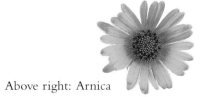

Above right: Arnica

HAY FEVER AND OTHER ALLERGIES

Over the last 20 or 30 years there has been an enormous increase in allergies, which might be better described as an over-sensitivity of the body to substances that cannot be easily assimilated. Hay fever, eczema, asthma, irritable bowel disease, chronic fatigue and other chronic diseases have reached almost epidemic proportions.

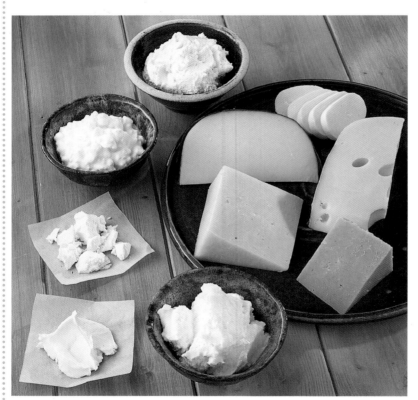

Above: Allergies, or over-sensitivity to certain foods, are becoming increasingly common. Dairy products and wheat-based foods seem to cause the most problems.

HOMEOPATHY AND CHRONIC DISEASE

No one knows precisely what causes these problems. There are undoubtedly a number of reasons. Toxicity overload is almost certainly one. The body simply cannot cope with the huge number of chemicals and drugs which it was not designed to absorb. Another reason is probably deficient nutrition. Many foods are now so over-processed that they do not contain sufficient minerals and vitamins to allow the body to function efficiently.

Homeopathy can often work wonders in correcting the many imbalances and weaknesses which result. Obviously, you should also take care to avoid toxic substances wherever possible, and eat a good, varied diet. The homeopathy needed to cure chronic ailments is complex and time-consuming, and beyond the scope of this book.

You will need help from a professional homeopath.

However, there is a certain amount you can do to alleviate the discomfort of acute hay fever symptoms.

HAY FEVER

Hay fever is rather a misnomer, for there are many other substances apart from hay which can trigger the well-known symptoms of watering eyes and runny nose, itchiness and sneezing. The problem may last for a few weeks, a few months or all year round, depending on the cause.

EUPHRASIA and *ALLIUM CEPA* are two of the most effective acute remedies. If the problem is centred in the eyes, with even the tears burning, Euphrasia is the remedy to use. However, if the nasal symptoms are worse, with constant streaming and an acrid discharge, then try Allium cepa.

Another remedy that is sometimes useful when there are constant burning secretions from the mucous membranes is *ARSENICUM*. This remedy also has a "wheezy" picture, so think of it when there is hay fever with asthmatic breathing, often worse at night.

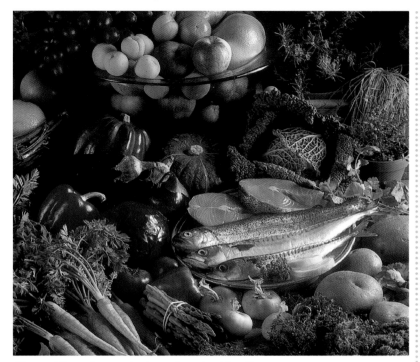

Above: There is no substitute for a healthy diet.

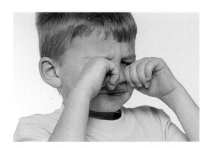

Above: The best remedy for hay fever, when the eyes are worst affected, is usually Euphrasia.

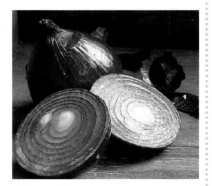

Above: Allium cepa.

TREATING BABIES AND CHILDREN

Children tend to respond very well to homeopathy and are a joy to treat. There is no substitute for constitutional treatment from an experienced professional homeopath, so that the overall immune system can be boosted as much as possible, but with a good stock of remedies there is much you can do at home in acute situations.

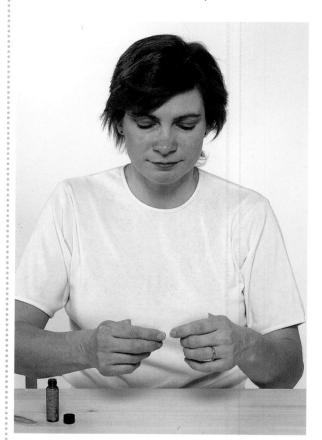

Above: For babies, it is essential to crush the tablet first.

CHILDREN AND HOMEOPATHY

The best start you can give a child is love and security, breast milk for as long as practical, a good varied diet, as few drugs as possible, and homeopathy. Young children often have dramatic acute conditions, such as fevers. Usually there is nothing to worry about if you are well informed, have professional support and have access to remedies. The dosage is the same as for adults, but remember to crush the pills first for babies.

TEETHING

The most widely used remedies for teething pains are *CHAMOMILLA* and *PULSATILLA*. Chamomilla is an "angry" remedy and suits bad-tempered babies best. These are the ones that drain you of sympathy because you have had so many sleepless nights and you feel so helpless. Only picking them up and carrying them around soothes them. Pulsatilla children respond differently – they are softer, weepy and invite your sympathy. They feel better and are soothed by being cuddled. They also need to be kept cool.

FEVERS

Many small children get fevers with very high temperatures, as they burn up infection in the most efficient way. Seek help if the fever goes on for more

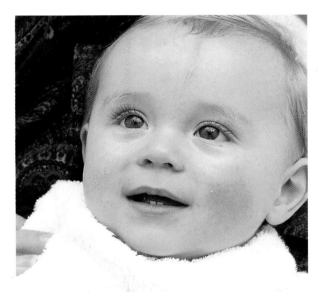

Above: For teething discomfort, Chamomilla or Pulsatilla are two of the most effective remedies.

than 24 hours, especially if there is a violent headache or drowsiness. ACONITE and BELLADONNA are the best general high fever remedies.

CROUP

This harsh, dry cough is very disturbing in small children, but usually sounds far worse than it is. There are three main remedies for croup. ACONITE can be used for particularly violent and sudden coughs, which are often worse at night. For harsh coughs that sound like sawing through wood, SPONGIA is the remedy. For a rattly chest with thick yellow-green mucus, possibly marked by irritability and chilliness, use HEPAR SULPH.

COLIC

This trapped wind (gas) and digestive pain can be very upsetting for a small baby. The baby may try to curl up to ease the pain, and warmth and gentle massage should help. MAG PHOS is a useful remedy to try.

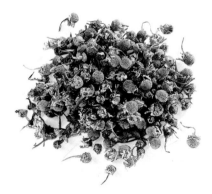

Above: The herb Chamomile, used in the remedy Chamomilla.

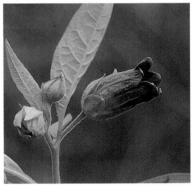

Above: Deadly nightshade, used in the remedy Belladonna.

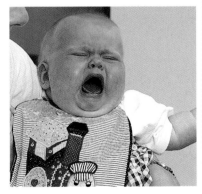

Above: For colicky babies, Mag Phos often soothes the pain as well as the nervous system.

WOMEN'S HEALTH PROBLEMS

A woman's weakest area often seems to be connected with her reproductive system and its associated hormones. The system is as delicate and intricate as a watch movement, but unfortunately it is often treated rather heavy-handedly by modern medicine. Many problems can be resolved by constitutional homeopathic treatment, as well as by dietary adjustments. For non-persistent conditions, homeopathic self-help will ease much distress.

ANAEMIA

Anaemia is usually caused by an iron deficiency and manifests itself through weakness, pallor and lack of stamina. The most vulnerable times are during pregnancy or after excessive blood loss due to heavy periods. Iron pills supplied by your doctor often severely upset the bowels, so gentler methods are preferable. Eat foods rich in iron and try organic iron preparations which can be obtained from health food shops. *FERRUM PHOS* should also be used daily.

CYSTITIS

Many women are familiar with the burning agony of urinating when they have a bladder infection. Cranberry juice or sodium bicarbonate can often help. Two of the most useful remedies are *CANTHARIS* and *APIS*. Use Cantharis as a general remedy. Apis can be helpful when the last drops in urination hurt the most.

MASTITIS

Mastitis means inflammation of the breast and occurs commonly during breast-feeding. It can be painful but is not normally serious. Breast-feeding does not have to stop because of it. Homeopathy is usually very successful in curing the inflammation.

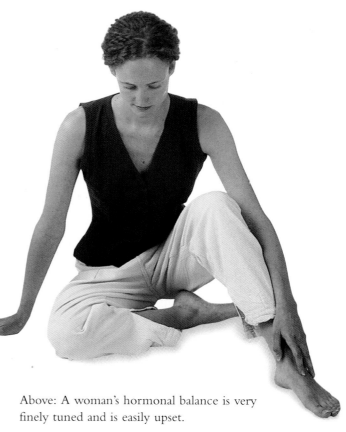

Above: A woman's hormonal balance is very finely tuned and is easily upset.

PHYTOLACCA has a special affinity with the breast area and is the most important remedy for the condition. The breast may feel lumpy as well as being swollen. The nipple may be cracked and particularly sensitive. If the breast looks very red and throbs painfully, *BELLADONNA* should be considered. *PULSATILLA* is also a remedy to think of when emotional issues are uppermost – especially when you feel unsupported and weepy.

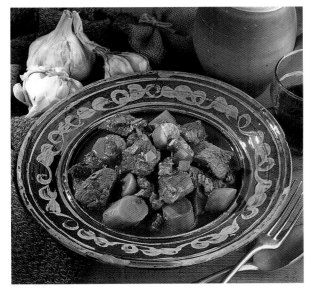

Above: Iron-rich foods include red meat, egg yolks, legumes, shellfish and parsley.

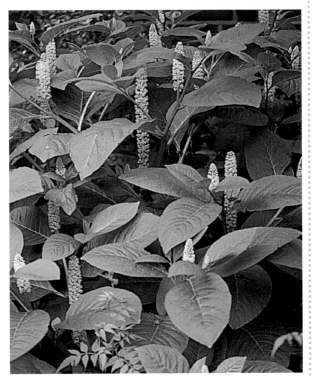

Above: One of the best all-round remedies for mastitis is Phytolacca.

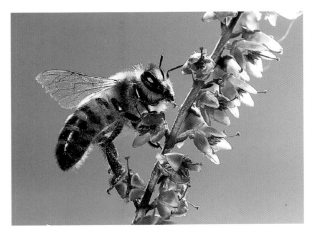

Above: The honey-bee, used in the remedy Apis.

PRE-MENSTRUAL TENSION (PMT)

Most women are familiar with the mood changes that arise just before an oncoming period. But for an unfortunate few, more extreme symptoms of depression, anger and weepiness can appear, sometimes as much as a week or more before the flow begins. A visit to a professional homeopath can often be of great benefit, but there are some remedies that you might try yourself at home to alleviate some of these very distressing symptoms.

PULSATILLA is an excellent remedy if weeping and the feeling of neediness is prominent. *SEPIA* should be used where there is anger and exhaustion, and even indifference towards your family. *LACHESIS* is helpful for the more extreme symptoms of violent anger, jealousy and suspicion.

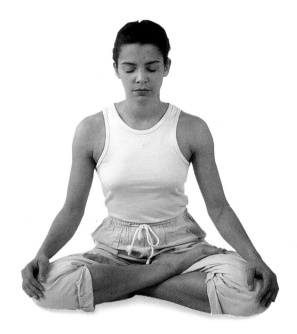

Above: Meditation can be an excellent way to relax the nervous system.

PERIOD PAINS

If your period pains are consistently bad, you will need to consult a homeopath. For occasional pains, there are a number of self-help remedies from which you can choose. The three PMT remedies mentioned above, *PULSATILLA, SEPIA* and *LACHESIS,* should be considered if the emotional symptoms described fit, and seem over-riding.

For pains that respond to warmth and make you want to curl up, *MAG PHOS* should be helpful. For very severe pains, with bad cramping, *VIBURNUM OPULUS* can be a great painkiller.

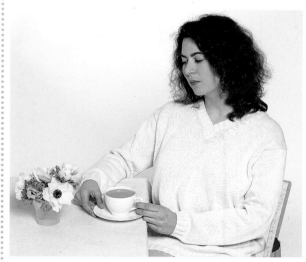

Above: PMT mood swings are not uncommon. Check your symptoms to find a remedy that might help.

MENOPAUSE AND HOT FLUSHES

Unfortunately, there is now a great tendency for doctors to treat the menopause as a disease, when it simply marks the end of a woman's childbearing years. Because of this there has been a great rush into Hormone Replacement Therapy (HRT). In fact, the symptoms of an out-of-balance menopause can usually be treated very successfully in a more natural way through nutrition and homeopathy. The remedies most often used are again *PULSATILLA, SEPIA* and *LACHESIS*. They can often be prescribed according to the personality and state of mind of the woman, as described previously for PMT.

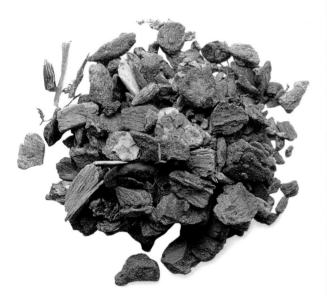

Above: Dried Cramp Bark, a herb used in the remedy Viburnum opulus.

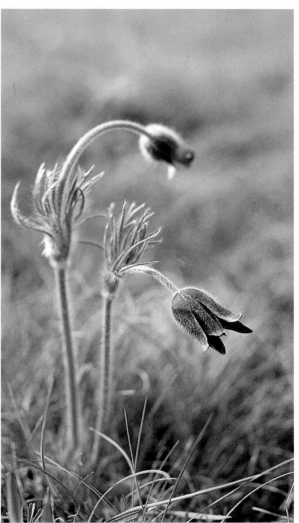

Above: The menopause is not an illness and does not have to be an ordeal. Pulsatilla is often used by homeopaths, with very good results.

EMOTIONAL ISSUES

We underrate at great risk the part our emotions play in our well-being. Much disease
can arise from the disharmony in our lives. This is even more likely if we are unable to express
our emotions and our feelings remain buried within us. Just as joy, laughter and the feeling of being
cared for can keep us in good health, the opposite feelings of sadness, hatred,
grief and insecurity are at the root of many illnesses.

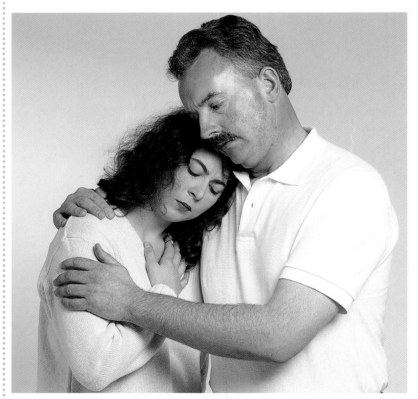

Above: The most useful remedy for emotional upsets, where you always
feel better for being comforted, is Pulsatilla.

EMOTIONAL TURMOIL

It is almost a daily occurrence for
a homeopathic practitioner to hear
words like "I've never really got
over my father's death," or "I've
never properly felt well since my
divorce." It is important for good
health not to allow such wounds
to fester too deeply. Homeopathy
can often assist both in chronic
conditions and in acute ones
where you feel you need help.

In any emotional situation
where you feel that you cannot
cope, always remember RESCUE
REMEDY. You can take it as often
as you like, alongside homeopathic
remedies if you wish.

GRIEF

IGNATIA is the number-one remedy
for acute feelings of sadness and
loss. It can calm both the hysterical and over-sensitive and those
who keep their grief bottled up.

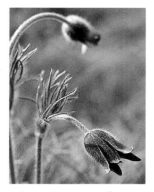

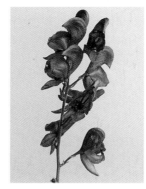

Above: A Pasque flower, used in Pulsatilla.

Above: Aconite.

Children and emotionally dependent people can be helped by *PULSATILLA*.

FRIGHT

ACONITE is the major remedy for helping people get over a shock or a terrifying experience.

ANTICIPATION

The worry over a forthcoming event such as an exam, appearing on the stage or meeting someone new can be very upsetting to some people. There are a number of remedies that can ease the anxiety and panic.

GELSEMIUM is best used when you start trembling with nerves and literally go weak at the knees. *ARG NIT* is a good all-round anxiety remedy, where there are symptoms of great restlessness. It also has a claustrophobic picture so could help with fear of flying or travelling by underground (subway). The panic often causes diarrhoea. Another anxiety remedy that can also affect the bowels is *LYCOPODIUM*. Strangely,

people who need Lycopodium often excel at the ordeals they have been worrying about, once they have gone through the panic barrier.

INSOMNIA

There can be many causes of sleeplessness: worry, habit, bad eating patterns and others. For the "hamster on the wheel" syndrome, where your mind is rushing around in never-ending circles, *VALERIAN* can be magical. For constant early waking, especially if you live too much on your nerves and eat too much rich food, try *NUX VOMICA*.

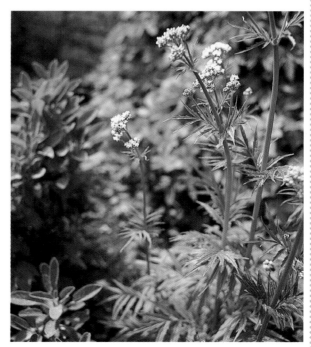

Above: The herb Valerian, used in the remedy Valeriana.

REMEDIES: THE MATERIA MEDICA

THERE ARE PERHAPS 2,000 remedies in the homeopathic Materia Medica, as it is called, although most of them are best left to the practitioner. However, there are a number of remedies that can be safely used by a lay person in low potencies for acute and first-aid purposes. The 42 remedies described in this chapter should be sufficient to cover most common problems.

Use this section to back up and confirm your choice from the remedies recommended for ailments in the previous chapter. If your choice still looks good, then you are probably on the right track. If it doesn't, consider one of the other remedies described for the ailment. Not every symptom of the remedy has to be present. Homeopaths use the expression "a three-legged stool": if the remedy covers three symptoms of the condition, then it is likely to be well indicated.

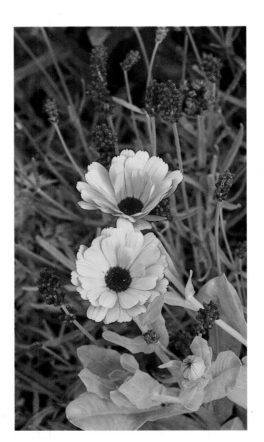

Above: Calendula flowers.

STORING HOMEOPATHIC REMEDIES

Keep your remedies in a cool dark place, away from strong smells and out of the reach of children. Homeopathic remedies are extremely safe, however, and even if a child swallows a number of pills, or even a whole bottle, there is nothing to worry about.

Right: A selection of materials that make up traditional homeopathic remedies. Clockwise from left: magnesium phosphate, flowers of sulphur, ground oyster shells, natural sponge, raw potash, potassium dichromate, viburnum opulus and iron phosphate.

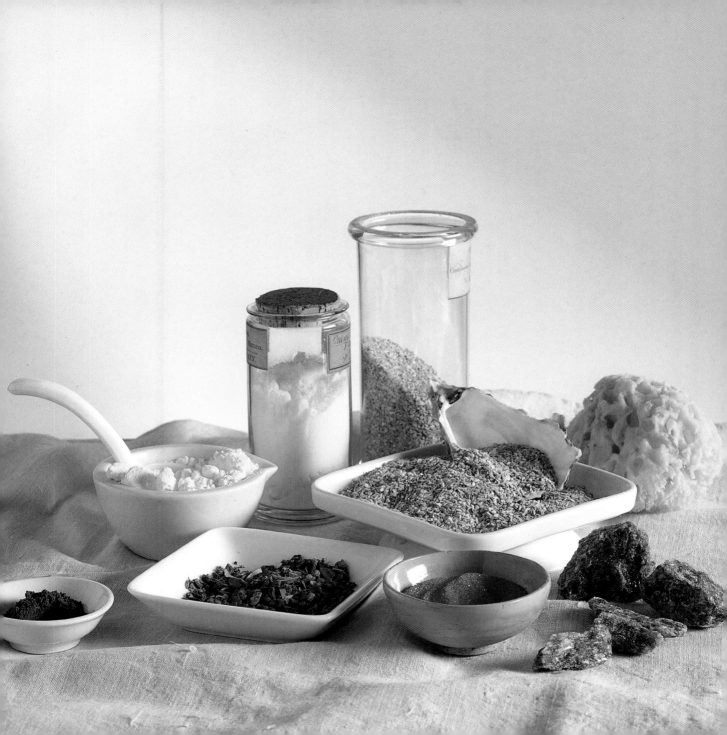

ACONITE

ACONITUM NAPELLUS

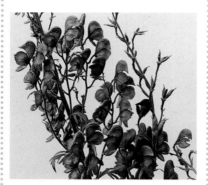

Monkshood, a beautiful yet poisonous plant with blue flowers, is native to mountainous areas of Europe and Asia. It is widely cultivated as a garden plant.

KEYNOTES
• Symptoms appear suddenly and violently, often at night.
• They may appear after catching a chill or after a fright.
• Fear or extreme anxiety may accompany symptoms.
• An important remedy for high fevers with extreme thirst and sweat.
• Major remedy for violent, dry croupy coughs.
• Best used at the beginning of an illness.

ALLIUM CEPA

ALLIUM CEPA

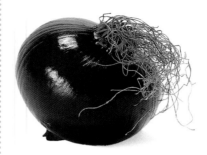

The remedy comes from the onion, whose characteristics are well known to anyone who has ever peeled one: it affects the mucous membranes of the nose, eyes and throat.

KEYNOTES
• Sneezing, often repeatedly, with a streaming nose.
• The nose and eyes burn and are irritated.
• Nasal discharge is acrid while the tears are bland.
• Major remedy for hay fever (when the nose is affected more than the eyes) and for colds.

ANT TART

ANTIMONIUM TARTARICUM

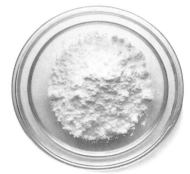

Ant tart is prepared from the chemical substance antimony potassium tartrate, traditionally known as tartar emetic. It affects the mucous membranes of the lungs.

KEYNOTES
• A wet, rattling cough from deep in the lungs, with shortness of breath and wheezing.
• Helps to bring up mucus from the lungs.

APIS

APIS MELLIFICA

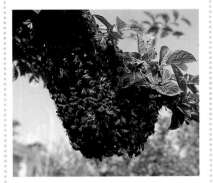

The remedy is prepared from the honey-bee. The well-known effects of its sting describe the remedy picture very well.

KEYNOTES
• A useful remedy after injuries, especially from bites or stings where there is swelling, puffiness and redness.
• The affected area feels like a water bag.
• Fever appears quickly and without thirst.
• The person is restless and irritable.
• The symptoms are often relieved by cool air or cold compresses.

ARG NIT

ARGENTUM NITRICUM

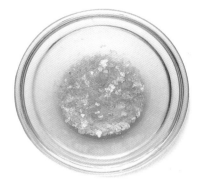

Silver nitrate, from which this remedy is derived, is one of the silver compounds used in the photographic process. It helps to soothe an agitated nervous system.

KEYNOTES
• Panic, nervousness and anxiety.
• Feeling worried, hurried and unsupported.
• Fears of anticipation, such as stage fright, exams, visiting the dentist, flying and many others.
• The nervousness may cause diarrhoea and wind (gas).

ARNICA

ARNICA MONTANA

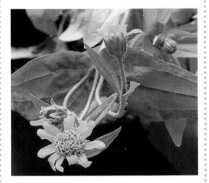

Arnica is a well-known herb with yellow, daisy-like flowers. It prefers to grow in mountainous areas. It has a special affinity with soft tissue and muscles, and is usually the first remedy to think of after any accident. Where there is bruising but the skin is not broken, use Arnica cream. (When the skin is broken, use Calendula or Hypercal cream instead.)

KEYNOTES
• The most important remedy for bruising.
• Shock following an accident.
• Muscle strains after strenuous or extreme exertion.

ARSENICUM

ARSENICUM ALBUM

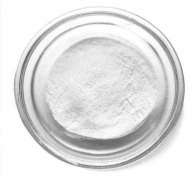

Arsenic oxide is a well-known poison. However, used as a home-opathic remedy it is extremely safe and works especially well on the gastro-intestinal and respiratory systems.

KEYNOTES
• Vomiting, diarrhoea, abdominal and stomach cramps.
• It is often the first remedy to try for food poisoning.
• Asthmatic, wheezy breathing, often worse at night. Head colds with a runny nose.
• Chilliness, restlessness, anxiety and weakness accompany the other symptoms.
• Warmth gives great relief in most ailments.

BELLADONNA

ATROPA BELLADONNA

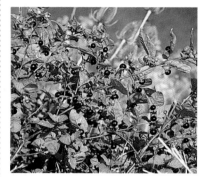

The remedy Belladonna is pre-pared from deadly nightshade, whose poisonous berries are best avoided. However, they produce a wonderful medicine which is one of the most important fever and headache remedies.

KEYNOTES
• Violent and intense symptoms appearing suddenly.
• Fever with high temperature, little thirst and burning, dry skin.
• The face or the affected part is usually bright red.
• Throbbing pains, especially in the head area.
• The pupils may be dilated and over-sensitive to light.

BRYONIA

BRYONIA ALBA

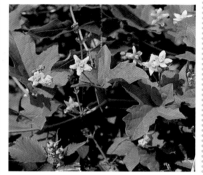

Bryonia is prepared from the roots of white bryony, a climbing plant found in hedgerows throughout Europe. The roots are enormous and store a great deal of water. Bryonia patients seem to lack "lubrication".

KEYNOTES
• The symptoms tend to develop slowly.
• Dryness marks all symptoms: in the mouth, membranes and joints.
• Extreme thirst.
• The condition feels worse for the slightest motion and better for firm pressure.
• Bryonia coughs are dry and very painful.
• The person is irritable.

CALENDULA

CALENDULA OFFICINALIS

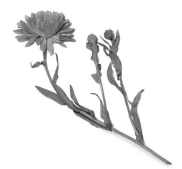

Calendula has long been known to herbalists as a major first-aid remedy for injuries. It is prepared from the common marigold, and the simplest way to use it is as a cream. Sometimes it is combined with Hypericum and the combination is known as Hypercal. You can use this cream on all cuts, sores and open wounds. (For bruises where the skin is not broken, use Arnica cream.)

Calendula is a natural antiseptic and keeps the injury free of infection, as well as speeding up the healing process.

IPECAC

CEPHAELIS IPECACUANHA

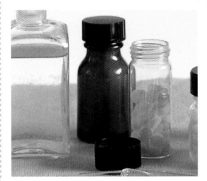

Ipecacuanha is a small South American shrub. The remedy works mainly on the digestive and respiratory tracts and the outstanding symptom is nausea, whatever the ailment.

KEYNOTES
• Persistent nausea, not helped by vomiting.
• Coughs accompanied by nausea.
• Morning sickness in pregnancy.
• Asthma or wheeziness with nausea.
• "Sick" headaches.

COCCULUS

COCCULUS ORBICULATUS

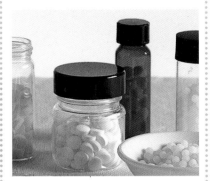

The remedy is prepared from the Indian cockle, a plant that grows along the coasts of India. It profoundly affects the nervous system and can strengthen a weakened and exhausted system. Because it can also cure nausea and dizziness, it is an important remedy for travel sickness, whether on a boat, plane or in a car.

KEYNOTES
• Nausea, vomiting, and dizziness, as in travel sickness.
• Exhaustion and nervous stress, perhaps due to lack of sleep.

DROSERA

DROSERA ROTUNDIFOLIA

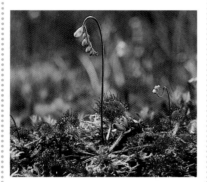

Drosera is a remedy prepared from an extraordinary insectivorous plant, the round-leaved sundew. Drosera affects the respiratory system and is an important cough remedy.

KEYNOTES
- Deep, barking coughs.
- Prolonged and incessant coughs returning in periodic fits or spasms.
- The cough may be so severe that it results in retching or vomiting.

EUPATORIUM

EUPATORIUM PERFOLIATUM

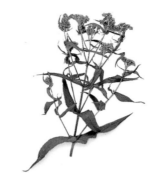

Eupatorium is a North American herb found growing in marshy places. Its common name, boneset, gives a clue to its use. Whatever the other symptoms, the bones usually ache. It is largely used as a flu remedy.

KEYNOTES
- Flu-like symptoms, with aching all over, but pains that seem to have lodged deep in the bones.
- There may be a painful cough, sometimes with nausea.

EUPHRASIA

EUPHRASIA OFFICINALIS

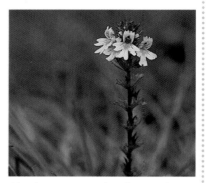

Also known as eyebright, Euphrasia has long been known as a remedy with a specific application to the eyes. It is a very pretty little meadow plant with colourful flowers that open wide only in sunshine.

KEYNOTES
- Eyes that are sore, red and inflamed.
- The eyes water with burning tears.
- In cases of hay fever, the symptoms are sneezing, itching and a runny nose, but the eyes are most affected.

FERRUM PHOS

FERRUM PHOSPHORICUM

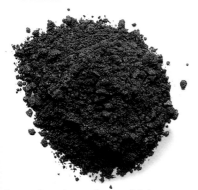

Iron phosphate, from which Ferrum phos is prepared, is a mineral that balances the iron and oxygen in the blood. It is a tissue salt that can be used as a tonic in weak anaemic patients.

KEYNOTES
• Flu and cold symptoms that are not well defined.
• Weakness and tiredness.
• General anaemia: the remedy can be very useful for women with heavy periods or during a pregnancy.

GELSEMIUM

GELSEMIUM SEMPERVIRENS

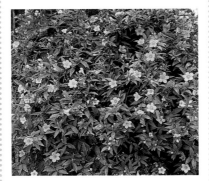

The remedy is prepared from a North American plant known as yellow jasmine. It acts specifically on the muscles, motor nerves and nervous system, and is probably the most important acute remedy for flu.

KEYNOTES
• Aching, heavy muscles which will not obey the will.
• Tiredness, weakness, shivering and trembling.
• Fever with sweating but little thirst.
• Headaches concentrated at the back of the head.
• Anticipation: the muscles tremble with fear at the thought of, or during, an ordeal.

HEPAR SULPH

HEPAR SULPHURIS CALCAREUM

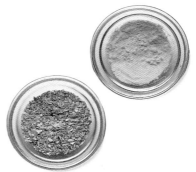

The remedy was developed by Hahnemann himself from calcium sulphide, which is made by heating flowers of sulphur and the lime of oyster shells together. It strongly affects the nervous system and is good in acute septic states (infected areas) and in respiratory system problems.

KEYNOTES
• Extreme irritability and over-sensitivity.
• Coldness, especially around the head.
• Hoarse, dry coughs with yellow mucus, croup.
• Abscesses and boils that contain a lot of pus and are slow to heal.
• Heavy perspiration.

HYPERICUM

HYPERICUM PERFORATUM

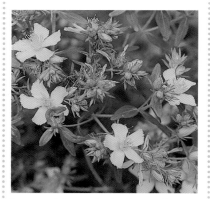

Prepared from the herb St John's Wort, Hypericum is primarily an injury remedy working particularly on areas rich in sensitive nerves: fingers, toes, lips, ears, eyes, and the coccyx at the base of the spine. Use Hypericum instead of Arnica for bruising in such sensitive areas, although Arnica may also work well.

KEYNOTE
• Pains are often felt shooting up the limbs, along the tracks of the nerves.

IGNATIA

IGNATIA AMARA

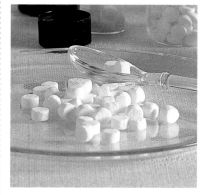

Ignatia is prepared from the seeds of a tree, the St Ignatius bean, which grows in South East Asia. It is a major "grief" remedy and strongly affects the emotions.

KEYNOTES
• Sadness and grief following emotional loss.
• Changeable moods: tears following laughter, or hysteria.
• Suppressed emotions, when the tears won't come.
• Pronounced sighing following a period of anxiety, fear or grief.

KALI BICH

KALI BICHROMICUM

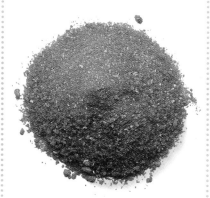

The source of Kali bichromicum, potassium dichromate, is a chemical compound involved in many industrial processes, such as dyeing, printing and photography. It especially affects the mucous membranes of the air passages and is an important sinusitis remedy.

KEYNOTES
• Thick, strong, lumpy green discharges from the nasal passages or mouth.
• Headaches in small spots as a result of catarrh.
• Dry cough with sticky, yellow-green mucus.

LACHESIS

LACHESIS MUTA

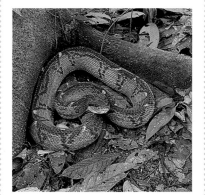

Lachesis is prepared from the venom of the bushmaster snake native to South America. Generally it is a chronic remedy best left in the hands of professional homeopaths, but it does have an acute use in treating sore throats and menstrual problems.

KEYNOTES
• Sore throats, much worse on the left side.
• Painful throats where liquids are more difficult to swallow than solids.
• Menstrual pains and tension improve when the flow starts.
• Hot flushes around the time of the menopause.

LEDUM

LEDUM PALUSTRE

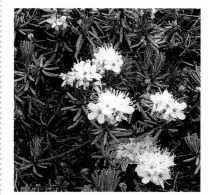

The small shrub known as marsh tea from which Ledum is derived grows in boggy places across the cold wastes of the Northern Hemisphere. It is primarily a first-aid injury remedy, where cold rather than warmth is found to be soothing.

KEYNOTES
• Puncture wounds such as from nails or splinters, bites and stings, whose pain is eased by cold compresses.
• Wounds that look puffy and feel cold.
• Injuries to the eye, which looks cold, puffy and bloodshot.

LYCOPODIUM

LYCOPODIUM CLAVATUM

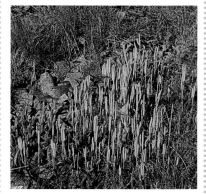

This remedy is prepared from the spores of club moss, a strange prostrate plant which likes to grow on heaths. It is mainly prescribed constitutionally for chronic conditions but it can be very helpful for digestive problems and sometimes for acute sore throats.

KEYNOTES
• Conditions that are worse on the right side or that move from the right to the left side of the body.
• Flatulence and pain in the abdomen or stomach.
• The problem is aggravated by gassy foods such as beans.
• The person may crave sweet things to eat.

CANTHARIS

LYTTA VESICATORIA

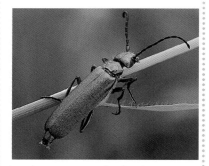

Cantharis is one of a few homeopathic remedies prepared from insects. It is derived from an iridescent green beetle commonly called Spanish fly. It is also known as the blister beetle, as it is a major irritant if handled. It has an affinity with the urinary tract.

KEYNOTES
• Cystitis - where there are intense, burning pains on urinating.
• Burns or burning pains generally, such as in sunburn or burns from hot pans.

MAG PHOS

MAGNESIA PHOSPHORICA

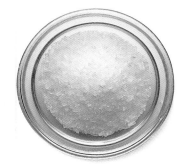

Magnesia phosphorica is one of the 12 tissue salts, as well as being a remedy, and works directly in easing tension in the nerves and muscles. It can therefore be an effective painkiller.

KEYNOTES
• Violent, cramping, spasmodic pains, often in the abdominal area.
• Pains are better for warmth, gentle massage or doubling up.
• Can help with colic, period pains, sciatica, toothache or earache.

CHAMOMILLA

MATRICARIA CHAMOMILLA

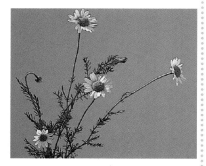

Chamomile is a member of the daisy family and grows wild throughout Europe and the US. It strongly affects the nervous system. The remedy is considered one of the most important medicines for the treatment of children: Aconite, Belladonna and Chamomilla are together known as the "ABC" remedies.

KEYNOTES
• Bad temper and irritability.
• Teething problems in angry babies.
• In cases of colic, the stools are usually offensive, slimy and green.
• Extreme sensitivity to pain.
• The child's temper is worse for being looked at or spoken to, and better for being rocked or carried.

MERCURIUS

MERCURIUS SOLUBILIS

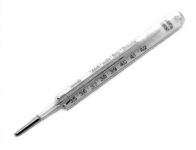

The name of this remedy is sometimes abbreviated to Merc sol. It is prepared from the liquid metal mercury. It is used in acute septic states (infected areas) where the glands and their secretions are particularly affected.

KEYNOTES
• Swollen and tender glands.
• Profuse sweating and increased thirst.
• The breath, sweat and secretions are usually offensive.
• The tongue looks flabby, yellow and coated.
• Fevers blow hot and cold.
• Irritability and restlessness.

PHOSPHORUS

PHOSPHORUS

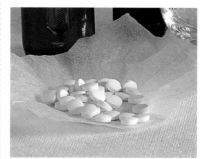

The element phosphorus is an important constituent of the body, particularly of the bones. It is normally used as a major constitutional remedy, but can be useful in some acute situations. These include digestive problems, with immediate vomiting once the food has warmed in the stomach, and constant diarrhoea as if a tap has been turned on. Phosphorus can also help with minor haemorrhages such as nosebleeds. A very useful application is for the "spacey" feeling that lingers too long after an anaesthetic.

KEYNOTE
• Suits people who are lively, open and friendly, but who are also occasionally nervous and anxious.

PHYTOLACCA

PHYTOLACCA DECANDRA

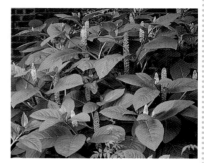

Phytolacca or poke-root is a plant that grows across the northern hemisphere. It is a glandular remedy that particularly affects the tonsils and mammary glands. Phytolacca is probably the most important remedy for mastitis.

KEYNOTES
• Sore throats that look dark and angry.
• Sore throats in which the pain feels like a hot ball and may extend to the ears.
• Swollen, tender breasts with hard lumps and cracked nipples.

PULSATILLA

PULSATILLA NIGRICANS

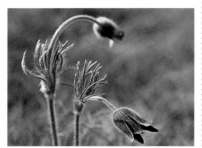

Pulsatilla is one of the most useful of acute remedies, as well as being a very important constitutional one. The remedy comes from the pasque flower and is also known as the weathercock remedy because it suits people whose moods and symptoms are constantly changing. For this reason, it is a wonderful remedy for small children.

KEYNOTES
• Tendency to be weepy and clingy, feeling unsupported.
• Suits people with gentle, sympathetic natures.
• Yellow-green discharge from the eyes or nose.
• Symptoms are helped by sympathy and fresh cool air.

RHUS TOX

RHUS TOXICODENDRON

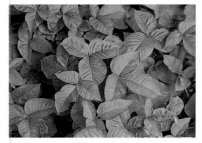

The remedy is prepared from poison ivy, native to North America. Its main use is in sprains, strains and swollen joints, but because of its itchy, rashy picture it can be a good remedy for illnesses such as chickenpox or shingles. It is also a useful remedy for acute rheumatism.

KEYNOTES
• Extreme restlessness with a red, itchy rash.
• Stiffness in the joints, which is eased by gentle motion.
• The symptoms are better for warmth and worse for cold, damp and over-exertion.

RUTA

RUTA GRAVEOLENS

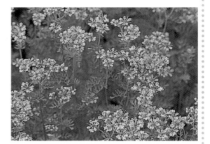

Ruta, or rue, is an ancient herbal remedy that has been called the herb of grace. It acts particularly on the joints, tendons, cartilages and periosteum (the membrane that covers the bones). It also has an affinity with the eyes.

KEYNOTES
• Bruises to the bones.
• Strains to the joints and connecting tissue, especially to the ankles and wrists.
• The symptoms are worse for cold and damp and better for warmth.
• Eye strain, with dim vision, from overwork.

SEPIA

SEPIA OFFICINALIS

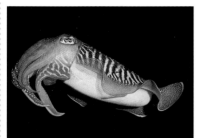

Sepia is a remedy prepared from the ink of the squid or cuttlefish. Normally its use should be left to the professional homeopath as it has a "big" picture (i.e. can be used in many circumstances), but because of its affinity with the female reproductive system it can be helpful in some menstrual problems.

KEYNOTES
• Suits tired, depressed, emotionally withdrawn people.
• Morning sickness in pregnancy, which is worse for the smell of food.
• Hot flushes during the menopause.
• Exercise may relieve the mental and emotional symptoms.

SILICA

SILICEA

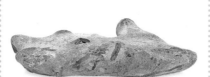

Silica is a mineral derived from flint. It is one of the 12 tissue salts, and its presence in the body aids the elimination of toxins. It can be used acutely in septic (infected) conditions to strengthen the body's resistance to continual infection and help to expel foreign bodies such as splinters. Silica can also help to bring lingering abscesses or boils to a head, or help the body to re-absorb pus harmlessly if appropriate.

KEYNOTES
• Suitable for symptoms that are slow to heal, or for people who feel the cold, or who lack stamina or vitality.
• Small-scale infections that seem to be turning septic or putrid, rather than healing.

SPONGIA

SPONGIA TOSTA

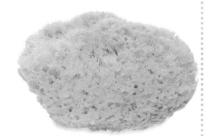

Spongia, as its name indicates, is a remedy prepared from the lightly roasted skeleton of the marine sponge. It works very well on the respiratory tract and is one of homeopathy's major cough remedies, and an important croup remedy for children.

KEYNOTES
• Dry spasmodic cough.
• The cough sounds like a saw being pulled through wood.

NUX VOMICA

STRYCHNOS NUX VOMICA

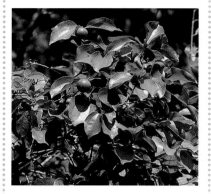

Nux vomica is prepared from the seeds of the poison nut tree of Southeast Asia. It is a remedy that has many uses in both chronic and acute situations, and is especially useful when the digestive system is involved.

KEYNOTES

• Nausea or vomiting after a rich meal, when the food remains undigested like a load in the stomach.
• A feeling that if only you could vomit you would feel better.
• An urge to pass a stool – but the results are unsatisfying.
• Heartburn with a feeling of sourness.
• Hangover headaches.

SYMPHYTUM

SYMPHYTUM OFFICINALE

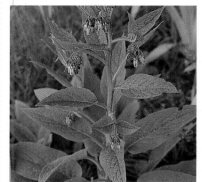

The remedy is prepared from the common herb comfrey. It is also known as knitbone, which indicates its main use in promoting the healing of broken bones. Use the remedy daily for several weeks after the bone has been set. Symphytum can also be used for injuries to the eyeball, such as after receiving the full force of a tennis ball directly in the eye.

KEYNOTES

• Speeds up the knitting or fusing together of bones.
• Injuries to the eyeball, such as being hit by a hard object.

VALERIAN

VALERIANA OFFICINALIS

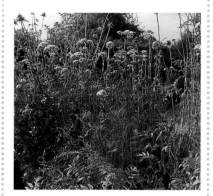

Valerian is a well-known herb whose overuse in the 19th century caused insomnia and overtaxation of the nervous system to the point of hysteria. Because of the principle "like cures like", very tiny doses such as those used in homeopathy can cure these very same problems. Valerian is an important remedy for sleeplessness. Take one pill about an hour before bedtime.

KEYNOTE

• Especially useful when the mind feels like a "hamster on a wheel".

VERBASCUM

VERBASCUM THAPSUS

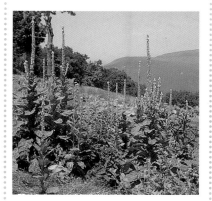

Verbascum is prepared from the great mullein, a common wayside herb. Its special use is in earaches, and it is best used as an oil. The remedy is especially helpful for children, who tend to suffer from ear infections more often than adults. Place a few drops of the oil in a warmed teaspoon and gently insert into the ear, with the child lying on one side.

KEYNOTE
• Earaches of all kinds, both in children and adults.

VIBURNUM OPULUS

VIBURNUM OPULUS

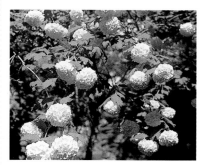

The guelder rose is widely distributed in woods and damp places throughout northern Europe and the US. It is also known as cramp bark and the homeopathic remedy, which is prepared from the bark, can be very helpful for period pains and spasmodic cramps.

KEYNOTE
• For severe cramping and muscle spasms.

RESCUE REMEDY

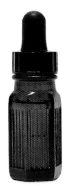

Although not strictly a homeopathic remedy – it is a combination of five of the Bach Flower essences – Rescue Remedy is such a wonderful medicine to have in your first-aid kit, it would be a real hardship to do without it. It usually comes in the form of a tincture, although it can also be bought as a cream. In any extreme crisis or shock, whether mental, emotional or physical, place a few drops on the tongue as often as necessary. Rescue Remedy can safely be used in conjunction with homeopathic remedies, or with other treatments or medicines.

INDEX

Picture Acknowledgements
The publishers gratefully acknowledge the following photographers and photographic agencies for permission to reproduce their photographs in this book:
A-Z Botanicals: p21tl/tr; p35mr; p41bm; p57tm; p60tr. **Heather Angel**: p57tl; p60tr; p61tr. **Bruce Coleman**: p43bl; p57tr; p62tm. **Mary Evans**: p6m. **Garden & Wildlife Matters**: p21ml/mr/b; p31br; p32br; p47br; p51tl; p52tm; p55tm; p62tr; p63tl/tm. **Lucy Mason**: p47tm; p50tl. **Papilio Photographic**: p54tl/tr. **Harry Smith**: p43br; p45r; p47tl; p52tr; p59tm/tr. **Warren Photographic**: p37br.

Key: t=top, m=middle, b=bottom; l=left, r=right

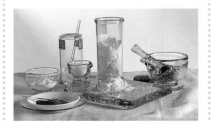

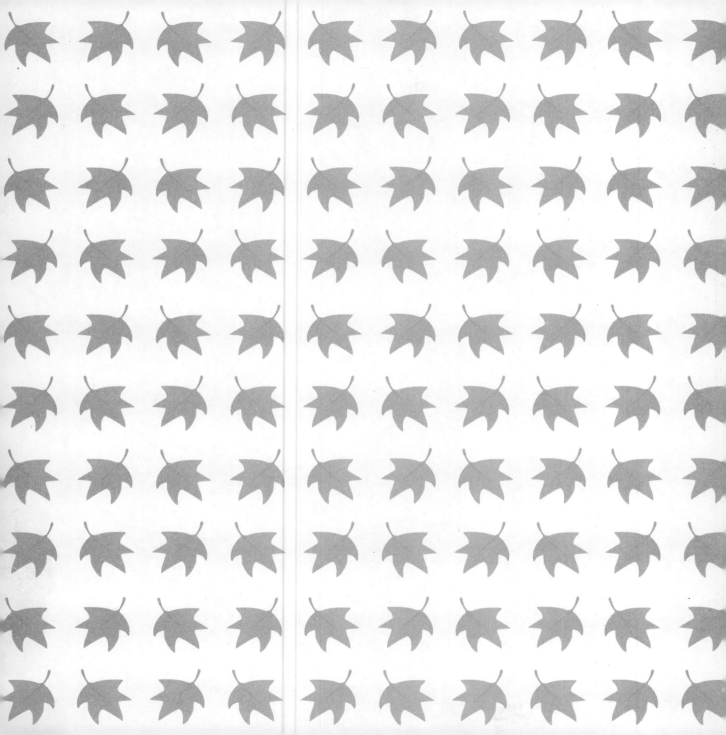